From the Editors of **Health** ®

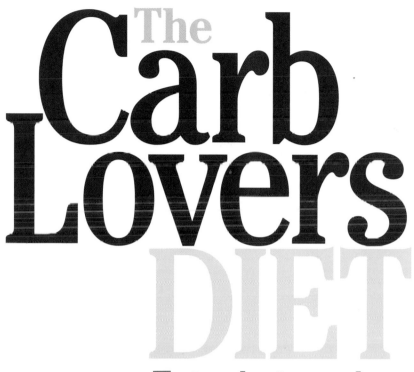

The Carb Lovers DIET

Eat what you love, get slim for life!

By **Ellen Kunes,** Editor in Chief,
and **Frances Largeman-Roth, RD,**
Health magazine

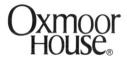

OXMOOR HOUSE®

ISBN-13: 978-0-8487-3370-4
ISBN-10: 0-8487-3370-3
Library of Congress Control Number: 2010925113
Printed in the United States of America
First Printing 2010

This book is intended as a general reference only, and is not to be used as a substitute
for medical advice or treatment. We urge you to consult your physician regarding any individual
medical conditions or specific health-related issues or questions.

Editor in Chief: Ellen Kunes
Creative Director: Ben Margherita
Executive Editor: Lisa Lombardi
Managing Editor: Faustina S. Williams
West Coast Editor: Jen Furmaniak (JB Talent)
West Coast Associate: Rachel Goldman (JB Talent)
Deputy Editor: Jennifer Brunnemer Slaton
Beauty and Fashion Editor: Colleen Sullivan
Beauty and Fashion News Editor: Jennifer Goldstein
Senior Editor: Su Reid-St. John
Senior Food and Nutrition Editor: Frances A. Largeman-Roth, RD
Medical Editor: Roshini Rajapaksa, MD
Associate Editors: Shaun A. Chavis, Susan Hall
Assistant Editor: Rozalynn S. Frazier
Office Manager: Stephanie Wolford
Editorial Assistants: Leslie Barrie, Caylin Harris, Kimberly Holland, Melanie Rud
Editorial Interns: Diana Cerqueira, Ashley Macha

ART DEPARTMENT
Design Director: José Fernandez
Senior Designer: Amanda Stevens

PHOTO DEPARTMENT
Photo Director: Marybeth Welsh Dulany
Contributing Photo Editors: Vanessa Griggs, Inna Khavinson
Art Production Assistant: Jamie Blair

COPY AND RESEARCH
Copy Chief: Tanya M. Hines-Wright
Research Editor: Michael Gollust
Assistant Copy Editor: Shannon Friedmann Hatch

PRODUCTION
Production Coordinator: Lauren A. Wade

TEST KITCHEN
Test Kitchen Director: Lori Powell
Recipe Contributor: Adeena Sussman

HEALTH.COM
Editorial Director: Ellen Kunes
Editor in Chief: Amy O'Connor
Executive Editor: Theresa Tamkins
Associate Editor: Ray Hainer
Assistant Editors: Mara Betsch, Kate Stinchfield

DEDICATION

Ellen:
Thanks so much to my wonderful husband, David, and my two amazing sons, Winston and Branch. You guys are the best, and I can't wait to take you out for a big carb-filled Italian dinner!

Frances:
A special thank you to my sweet husband, Jon, and daughter, Willa, for their patience and support and for trying all those carbo-licious recipes.

contents

acknowledgments

I'VE BEEN ON SOME TYPE OF DIET since I was 15 years old. Using a bit of (scary!) addition, that means for the past 36 years I've been counting calories, fasting, juicing, chewing gum, avoiding carbs, avoiding fat, avoiding sugar, and generally obsessing about my weight.

I know I'm not alone here: Weight control is something that *Health* magazine's and Health.com's 14 million readers obsess about, too. So we decided to dedicate ourselves to finding a way out of all this diet madness—and uncover a whole new way to eat. It has always been our dream to create a plan that would allow each and every one of us to relax and enjoy eating again.

I'm a *CarbLover* from way back…and I was *soooo* tired of feeling guilty about every slice of bread and each cup of pasta I ate. That's why I was excited when two years ago, *Health*'s amazing Food Editor, Frances Largeman-Roth, RD, and our in-house weight-loss guru, associate editor Shaun Chavis, told me the news about Resistant Starch, a type of carbohydrate researchers were really talking about: All their studies were showing that Resistant Starch could boost metabolism, curb cravings, lower cholesterol…it looked like this miracle carb could be the solution to our eternal diet problems. *Health*'s editors followed the studies, and talked to the experts, and it soon became clear that the era of low-carb eating might soon be OVER! A new and better way of eating was about to dawn.

Here it is...in your hands, the product of voluminous and careful research and rigorous testing by everyone here at *Health*. As our one (and only!) weight-loss book, it was important to us that you be as thrilled with our diet plan as we are. This is truly a diet you can stick with—and enjoy—for the rest of your life.

Of course, many people helped create this groundbreaking plan:

First, a huge thank you to the whole *Health* staff, who worked so tirelessly on *CarbLovers,* all while putting out a great magazine and website: Shaun Chavis and Jennifer Slaton—you guys are simply amazing. And Amy O'Connor, editor in chief of Health.com: There would be no *CarbLovers* without your initiative and incredibly hard work! Also making it happen from *Health:* Dave Watt, Renee Tulenko Ben Margherita, Lisa Lombardi, Su Reid-St. John (thanks for that amazing workout!), Marybeth Welsh Dulany, Faustina Williams, Jen Furmaniak, Susan Hall, Rozalynn Frazier, Kimberly Holland, Michael Gollust, our incomparable medical editor Roshini Rajapaksa, MD, and Health.com's Mara Betsch, who, with Amy O'Connor, helped coordinate the fabulous online version of *CarbLovers*.

A huge thanks to Sylvia Auton and John L. Brown for being such wonderful supporters of *Health* and giving us all the tools we needed to create this book. Thanks, too, to the terrific editors of Time Home Entertainment Inc. and Oxmoor House: Richard Fraiman, Jim Childs, Susan Payne Dobbs, Sydney Webber, Tom Mifsud, Fonda Hitchcock, and Laurie Herr. Another round of thanks to our crack legal team: Rebecca Sanhueza, Michelle McHugh, and Helen Wan.

There are a number of other people who did incredible work helping us get this book to you: They include reporter/researcher Alisa Bowman; dietitians Dawn Jackson Blatner, RD, and Marissa Lippert, RD; and recipe developer extraordinaire Shea Zukowski. A special thank-you to Maxine Davidowitz for her brilliant *CarbLovers* design; to Scott Mowbray for helping us get going on the project; to José Perez for helping focus our efforts; and to Debra Richman, Heidi Krupp, and their teams for helping us spread the word so quickly and so well about the magic of *CarbLovers*.

Frances wants to give a huge thank-you to Rhonda Witwer at National Starch and Hope Warshaw, RD, for sharing their Resistant Starch knowledge. And a special thanks, too, from Frances to *Health*'s Leslie Barrie and Caylin Harris "for helping me keep my head on straight!"

And our deepest gratitude goes to those who lost big on *The CarbLovers Diet* and helped us fine-tune the diet so millions of you could experience the thrill of getting slim WHILE eating carbs. We couldn't have done it without you!

Ellen Kunes,
Editor in Chief, *Health* magazine

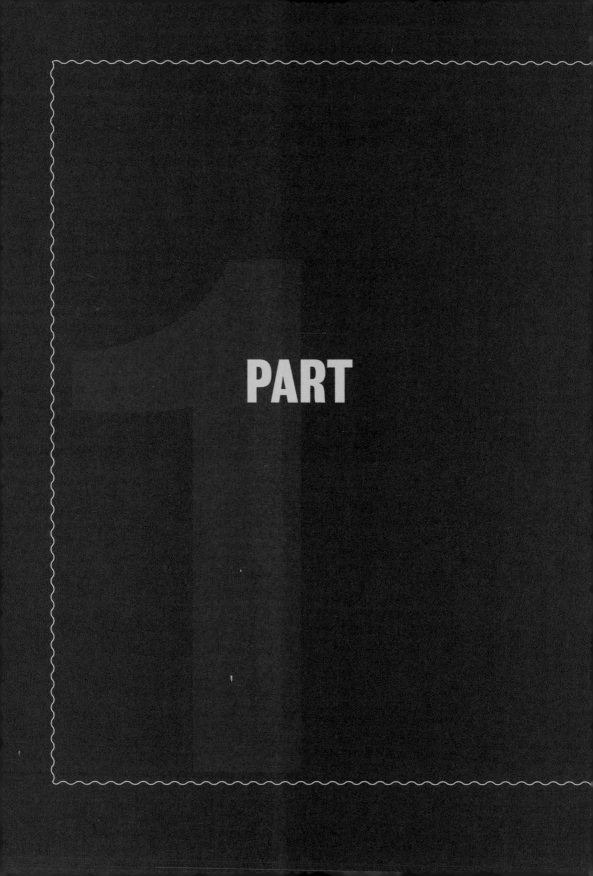

PART

Eat Carbs, Get Thin

Chapter 1

You Can Get and Stay Slim on Carbs...Really!

NOT SO LONG AGO, I was at one of my book club's potluck dinners: We'd been reading the best-selling memoir *Eat, Pray, Love,* so I brought an amazingly tasty pesto pasta salad to mark the fabulous Italian "Eat" section so lovingly detailed in the book. Then I watched as my six friends each took a tiny spoonful of my pasta dish—treating it like it was a nugget of plutonium on plates that they'd otherwise dutifully filled with sliced chicken breast (no gravy, of course!) and salad (dressing on the side, naturally!). After they devoured their morsels of pasta, they practically licked the spot on the plate where it had been. Then they proceeded to talk about how guilty they felt for eating even a forkful of carbs!

Carbo-phobia!

This "fear of carbs" is rampant: Almost every woman I know has it. We've learned to fear carbs because we've been told for more than 25 years that foods filled with carbohydrates make us gain weight. If you're like me, that means that you're afraid of eating toast with your eggs in the morning. You're afraid of a simple cheese sandwich. You're afraid of baked potatoes. You're afraid of pizza. You're afraid of pasta. Every time you eat one of these delicious basics of a happy, pleasure-filled life, you're overcome with guilt—and the conviction that you are now going to pile on the pounds. Fast.

Well, we, the editors of *Health* magazine, have big news for you. Trust me when I say that if you're carbo-phobic, it has to end right here, right now.

That's because there is new research—reliable, solid, groundbreaking research by the smartest minds in nutrition science right now—that reveals our old, beloved, carb-filled foods will NOT make us fat. Instead, they will actually make us THIN.

You Can Lose Weight on Carbs!

You're probably wondering—so what's changed? Maybe you're feeling whip-sawed once again by the diet experts. So let me tell you how we first learned about the new "carb-think" and why it inspired us not only to write about it in *Health* magazine, but also to create our very first weight-loss book.

Two years ago, one of my editors mentioned some new research on carbo-hydrates that she heard at a scientific conference in Philadelphia. The nutrition experts there seemed very excited about it, she said. "Would you take a look at the research?"

So I did—and what I read reversed a lifetime of assumptions I had about what makes people lose weight and keep it off.

The most astonishing studies were conducted by scientists at The University of Colorado Health Sciences Center for Human Nutrition, in Denver, along with a team of international researchers.[1] They uncovered new evidence that revealed eating the right carbs is the best way to get *and* stay slim.[2] These exciting new studies showed that certain carb-rich foods act as metabolism boosters and

"I watched as my six friends
each took a tiny spoonful of
my pasta dish—treating it like
it was a nugget of plutonium."

appetite suppressants in your body. I'll lay out all the important details of what the researchers uncovered in Chapter 2, but the bottom line is that rather than making you fat and bloated, carbs can actually do this:

- shrink fat cells, especially in your belly
- boost fat burning
- preserve muscle mass
- curb cravings
- keep you feeling full longer than other foods
- control blood sugar
- lower cholesterol and triglycerides

Around the same time, other research centers (including those at The University of South Carolina, The University of Minnesota, Louisiana State University, and even prestigious centers in Australia, Great Britain, and Denmark) were coming to similar conclusions.[3, 4]

Perhaps the most surprising piece of research was a large-scale look into the eating patterns that determine whether people will be fat or skinny over the course of a lifetime. **This multicenter study of 4,451 people found something stunning: It concluded that the slimmest people ate the <u>most</u> carbs (in the form of whole grains, fruits, and vegetables), and the chubbiest people ate the fewest carbs.**[5] The researchers even found that your odds of getting and staying slim are best when carbs comprise up to 64 percent of your total calorie intake, or 361 grams a day. That's the equivalent of several baked potatoes (a food you've probably avoided for decades).

None of the low-carb diets I've ever tried allowed me to eat that many carbs. Most of the diets I've tried in the past 25 years have limited the carb count to less than 30 percent of total calories allowed. A few even kept the total to just 10 percent of total calories.

All of this means that if you're a longtime low-carb dieter and you eat double or even triple the amount of carbs you've been allowing yourself—you won't get fat. In fact, you'll finally be eating the way the slimmest people have been eating all along!

Getting Ready To Lose Weight on Carbs

If you've been convinced for years that eating carbs will make you fat, it's going to take time for you to adjust to the new reality that they are the best things that ever happened to your waistline.

There's something else I have to tell you right now before we begin. And that is, although this is a diet plan that will show you how to live a life full of wonderful, soul-satisfying carbs, being a *CarbLover* does not mean you get to stuff yourself with bagels and cookies all day. What you'll be doing on this plan is increasing your total intake of carbs and upping the percentage of a type of carb called "Resistant Starch" in your diet. Resistant Starch is a kind of carbohydrate getting lots of attention in scientific circles these days. Yes, it has a strange name, but it's called that for a very good, and very important, reason: It resists digestion.

This is a great boon for weight loss (and your overall health) because Resistant Starch doesn't get absorbed into the bloodstream in the small intestine like other foods—but it does create a chain reaction in your body, literally shrinking fat cells, preserving muscle, stoking your metabolism, and making you feel fuller, longer.

Ask the carb pro

Frances Largeman-Roth, RD

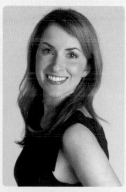

Q. What's the best way to get ready to start *The CarbLovers Diet?*

A. You want to start this new diet feeling energetic and clearheaded. So instead of a last-ditch binge, hold a kitchen reorganization party. Gather all of your Power Pantry items (page 41). Store your grains, and mark your containers. Plan your recipes for the week, and prep some of what you'll be eating the following day. And get a good night's sleep!

Studies show that adding a little Resistant Starch to your to morning meal will shift your body into fat-melting mode so that you burn nearly 25 percent more calories a day. Meanwhile, you'll eat about 10 percent fewer calories—simply because you're not as hungry (foods containing Resistant Starch are quite filling, so you end up eating less overall.)[6]

But here's the best news of all: Resistant Starch-filled foods aren't those exotic, super-expensive ingredients you can only get via mail-order from Hawaii. They're right here, at your local supermarket. They are bread, cereals, potatoes (even potato chips!), and bananas (we'll give you a more detailed list on pages 32–33). In other words, the foods with the highest Resistant Starch levels just happen to be delicious, affordable, and satisfying—and you can find them at any grocery store. These are the real foods you've been hungry for—and don't ever have to be deprived of again.

Lose Fast on The 7–Day *CarbLovers* Kickstart Plan

The *CarbLovers* Diet begins with a 7-Day *CarbLovers* Kickstart Plan (starting on page 59) developed by two top dietitians. We know how hard it may be to allow yourself, after years of denying yourself delicious carbs, to start eating them again. That's why our 7-Day *CarbLovers* Kickstart Plan helps you transition to your new world of eating and feeling satisfied. On it, you'll quickly knock off up to 6 pounds and reduce belly bloat, all while feeling full, in control, and super-energized!

Drop More on The 21–Day *CarbLovers* Immersion Plan

After you've tasted success on the 7-Day *CarbLovers* Kickstart Plan, you're ready for the life-changing 21-Day *CarbLovers* Immersion Plan (starting on page 73). This is the heart and soul of *The CarbLovers Diet*. It's basically a plan that gets you back to the way you used to eat before you made carb deprivation a way of life. The Plan itself is a breeze. Our experts did all the calculations for you, so all you have to do is eat and enjoy.

Think of the 21-Day *CarbLovers* Immersion Plan as a roadmap to the future— an incredibly easy-to-follow set of basic eating rules, daily menus, grab-and-go foods, and delicious recipes anyone can make, enjoy, and share with others. Don't feel like cooking? No problem. We've got more than 100 quick bites that work with *The CarbLovers Diet*, too.

Together, we'll wade into virgin territory, which will soon find you: shopping for new ingredients (or yummy grab-and-go items) at the grocery store; cooking up simple, delicious recipes; ordering what you want at your favorite restaurants; and enjoying meals with friends and family—all while getting and staying slim. We'll support your new eating life with tips, recipes, and clear-cut meal plan that will change your relationship with food and keep you from ever going hungry again. By the end of this three weeks, you'll have lost up to another 6 pounds!

Becoming a *CarbLover* for Life

In Chapter 8, you'll find proven get-to-goal strategies, including ideas for helping you reach your goal weight even faster if you make some small tweaks to your lifestyle. Exercise, smarter sleep habits, and cooking tricks can speed up weight loss while you're still enjoying carbs.

As you lose weight, our dietitians—as well as real women who've already successfully lost weight on *CarbLovers*—will encourage you every step of the way. If you have a little "I can't believe I ate that muffin!" panic attack, we're there too…with real-life advice from women who've lost big, as well as experts who can reassure you that the road map to lasting weight loss is the very one you are on. Finally, when you've reached your goal weight, we'll tell you how to stay as slim as you want to be, forever (starting on page 251).

So get ready for the best—and only—diet plan you'll ever need. Do you love making special meals for friends and family? Have we got some great recipes for you! You can also have a great social life while on *CarbLovers:* Enjoy a glass of wine (and some amazing pasta salad!) with your book club! Or how about tacos (pages 104 and 172) after work with co-workers? You can create decadent desserts your family will love, like our *CarbLovers* Dark Chocolate & Oat Clusters (page 213). In fact, in Chapter 7, you'll find over 75 easy, tasty recipes for nearly every eating moment of your life.

We've also built an easy-to-navigate website. At **carblovers.com,** you'll find even more recipes, meet other dieters, and get real-time advice from the same experts who helped create this groundbreaking plan. Turn the page, and start eating what you love, and at the very same time, start dropping that stubborn 15, 35, 100 pounds—or more! Get ready to feel satisfied, happy, and oh-so-slim. Get ready for your fabulous new life as a *CarbLover*!

"I Lost Weight on *CarbLovers*"

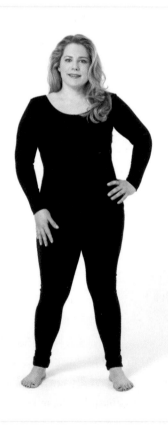

ALI HOCART

Age: 39

Height: 5'3"

Weight before: 164

Weight after: 140

Pounds lost: 24

Biggest success moment: I've gone from someone people called "pretty but chunky" to "the incredible shrinking woman." It feels great!

Biggest challenge: On my previous diet attempts, I failed in silence. This time, I asked for support and encouragement—and got it.

Favorite recipe: I'm a real bread-and-cheese person, so my favorites were the Sharp Cheddar & Egg on Rye (page 134) and the Tomato & Mozzarella Melt (page 136).

AFTER

I struggled to lose weight for years. Even though I was a serial dieter, somehow I could never stay slim. I tried diets with packaged foods and meals like Jenny Craig and The Zone, as well as high-protein plans. Inevitably I'd get discouraged, quit, regain the weight—and sometimes I'd put on even more! I was so frustrated that I committed to a serious exercise routine. But even after months of working out with a trainer, it became clear that exercise alone wasn't going to be enough. That was a difficult reality to face.

CarbLovers was my last chance, so I decided to give it a try. The first thing I did was give up diet sodas and prepared diet-food junk. Then I started cooking from scratch and taking my lunch to work instead of eating out. For the first time in forever I was eating whole, real food—and feeling my taste buds come alive again!

I like how *CarbLovers* lets you eat what you want, but teaches you to manage your cravings. For example, I love rich chocolate cakes and pastries. So I made up something that reminds me of a chocolate croissant: I sprinkle a tablespoon of dark chocolate chips on a corn tortilla (Resistant Starch!), put it in the broiler for 45 seconds, and roll it up. It's amazing!

After just 12 weeks on *CarbLovers,* I'm halfway to my goal. People tell me my skin looks better. My confidence has improved dramatically. I'm so excited about getting dressed in the morning and being able to shop for clothes again.

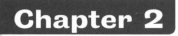

Chapter 2

The Truth About Low-Carb Diets
(and Why You Gotta Eat Carbs to Be Slim)

FINALLY, THE TRUTH COMES OUT: Those low-carb diets (all of them!) you've been trying to follow for the last 1, 7, even 10 years? According to experts, in the long run, low-carb diets just don't work! Now, it's true that low-carbohydrate, high-protein plans can help you lose weight in the short term. Over the past 10 years, I've lost 20 pounds…and then gained that same 20 pounds back—maybe five times!—on a variety of low-carb plans. My experience, say diet researchers, is all too common. In fact, nutrition researchers say that limiting your carbs just doesn't work over the long haul because we are hardwired to crave carbohydrates.

And that spells carb-fueled BINGES. With all those binges, it is absolutely inevitable that you'll gain back most, if not all, of the weight you lost on that low-carb diet in the first place. Want to know a few more reasons why you need to steer clear of the low-carb way of life? Read on.

5 Truths About Low-Carb Diets

1. Low-carb diets make you feel sad and stressed!

Snapping at your husband and kids? Yelling at the driver in front of you who just isn't going fast enough? You might want to blame your carb-deprivation. A recent study by Australian researchers, published in the *Archives of Internal Medicine,* followed 106 dieters for a year. Half ate a carb-rich diet; the others followed a low-carb diet. After a year, the carb-eaters felt happier, calmer, and more focused than the carb-deprived group, who reported feeling stressed out.[1] Another study at The University of Toronto found that dieters who restricted carbs for just three days reported feeling more depressed than before restricting them.[2] The reason? Carbs boost mood-regulating, stress-reducing chemicals in the brain, and high-protein, fatty foods may deplete them, says Grant Brinkworth, PhD, lead researcher of the Australian study.

2. Low-carb diets make you fatter, not thinner!

The stress and depression low-carb dieters feel eventually derails their best efforts to stay slim. That's because stress produces high levels of hormones, like cortisol, which boost your appetite and can lead to bingeing, says obesity researcher Elissa Epel, PhD, associate professor in the Department of Psychiatry at The University of California, San Francisco.

3. Low-carb diets are not sustainable!

It's one thing to tough out a low-carb diet for six weeks or even six months. It's another to do it for a lifetime, and studies show that people have a harder time sticking with low-carb rather than high-carb diets. In a 2009 Israeli study of 322 dieters, only 78 percent of those on low-carb plans stuck with their diets for the long term (up to two years), while nearly 90 percent of those who ate a more balanced-in-carbs diet were still going strong after two years.[3] "It's hard to consistently follow a diet that is very low in carbs or very high in carbs," says weight-loss researcher Anwar T. Merchant, ScD, DMD, associate professor of epidemiology and biostatistics at The University of South Carolina.

"Carbs boost mood-regulating, stress-reducing chemicals in the brain."

4. Low-carb diets bloat your belly!

Think carbs are the reason you can't zip your pants? Think again. According to the National Institute of Digestive Diseases, belly bloat is one of the key symptoms of constipation. And constipation is a common side effect of a low-carb diet. In one study, as many as 68 percent of participants on a low-carb diet complained of constipation.[4] That's compared to just 30 percent of the general non-dieting population and 35 percent of dieters who ate more carbs.

5. Low-carb diets make you feel deprived!

Any dieter who has managed to stick to a very low-carb diet for any length of time knows that they start craving carbs. And it's not your imagination. According to research at The University of Toronto, carb deprivation leads directly to carb bingeing. In one study of 89 women, half restricted the amount of carbs they ate, while the other half did not. After three days, when both groups were served a breakfast and told to eat all that they wanted, the women on the low-carb diet stuffed themselves with calorie and fat-laden carbs (like croissants), while the women who had been on diets with a balanced amount of carbs continued to follow their diets.[5] Bottom line: If you stop eating carbs, it's almost impossible not to binge on them when given the opportunity.

The Amazing News About Carb-Rich Diets

While there is now solid research that reveals low-carb diets are destined to fail, there is just as much evidence—in fact, even more evidence—that eating a diet packed with the right kind of carbs is *the secret to getting and staying slim for life.*

When we talk about the right kind of carb, what we mean is the kind of carbohydrate called Resistant Starch. Nearly 200 important studies conducted at respected universities and research centers around the world have shown Resistant Starch to be an extraordinary, 100-percent natural appetite suppressant and metabolism booster that will change the way you think about dieting forever.

Resistant Starch is a carbohydrate that *resists digestion*. It's found in ordinary foods you already eat and can buy at any supermarket. All of this solid research shows that consuming more of this special carbohydrate helps you:

- eat less
- burn more calories
- feel more energized and less stressed
- steady blood sugar levels

The science behind Resistant Starch is truly incredible: We explain exactly how it works later in this chapter.

But first, because we know you've been conditioned for so long to think of bread and pasta and rice and potatoes as bad-for-you foods, we want to explain to you all the reasons why getting carbs back into your diet isn't only good for you…it's absolutely essential if you want to lose weight and keep it off for the rest of your life.

The top weight-loss experts we've talked to all agree. "There are three things that dictate success with losing weight and maintaining that weight loss," says veteran weight-loss researcher Larry Tucker, PhD, a professor of exercise science at Brigham Young University in Provo, Utah: "The diet has to be healthy, it has to be effective, and it has to be sustainable. It can't be something that you think you can tough out for a few weeks or a few months. It has to be something that eventually becomes a lifestyle." And that lifestyle, explains diet researcher Dr. Merchant, *must* include a healthy helping of foods like bread, potatoes, fruits, and vegetables. "The good news is that people who maintain an optimal body weight are not following a very low-carbohydrate diet or a very high-carbohydrate diet," he says. "They are eating regular, balanced meals that include carbs."

There's barely enough room in this book to list the solid, evidence-based reasons you must get carbs back in your life if you are ever to achieve the sleek, slim look you've been wanting for so long. Here are a few, though, that we thought you should absolutely commit to memory.

9 Reasons You Need Carbs in Your Life

1. Eating carbs makes you thin for life!

As I mentioned in Chapter 1, a recent multicenter study of thousands of people found that the slimmest people also ate the most carbs, and the chubbiest ate the least. The researchers concluded that your odds of getting and staying slim are best when carbs comprise up to 64 percent of your total calorie intake, or 361 grams a day. That's the equivalent of several baked potatoes (a food we bet you've been afraid to eat for decades).[6] None of the low-carb diets I've ever tried allowed you to eat that many carbs. In fact, most low-carb diets limit you to fewer than 30 percent of total calories, or 150 grams a day. And some low-carb diets have almost no carbs at all: They have as little as just 10 percent of calories from carbs!

The CarbLovers Diet allows you to double, even triple your carb intake— compared to low-carb plans—so you can start eating the way the slimmest people have been eating all along.

2. Carbs fill you up!

Many carb-filled foods act as powerful appetite suppressants. They're even more filling than protein or fat. These special carbs fill you up because they are digested more slowly than other types of foods. The carbs in *The CarbLovers Diet* quickly trigger a sensation of fullness in both your brain and your belly. As a result, you stay satisfied longer—so much longer that you'll find that you eat less automatically. Research done at The University of Surrey in Great Britain found that consuming Resistant Starch in one meal caused study participants to consume 10 percent fewer calories (roughly 150 to 200 calories for the average woman) during the next day because they felt less hungry.[7]

3. Carbs curb your hunger!

These good-news carbs also raise levels of satiety hormones that tell the brain to flip a switch that stifles hunger and turns up metabolism. "High-fiber carbohydrates such as brown rice and grains allow you to eat to the point of satisfaction and still lose weight," says Tucker. "You can lose weight, and you don't have to be hungry at all."

4. Carbs control blood sugar and help prevent diabetes!

The right mix of carbs is the best way to control blood sugar and thus keep type 2 diabetes at bay. In one study done at the Beltsville Human Nutrition Research Center at the United States Department of Agriculture, participants who consumed a diet rich in the foods featured in *The CarbLovers Diet* were able to lower their post-meal blood sugar and insulin response by up to 38 percent.[8] *The CarbLovers Diet* lets you eat all the carbs you want, but we've combined them with other foods so that they don't cause a spike in your blood sugar. Instead, you'll be enjoying carbs that keep your blood sugar more balanced than traditional low-carb diets.

5. Carbs speed up metabolism!

The CarbLovers Diet is filled with carbohydrates that speed up your metabolism and your body's other natural fat-burners. As Resistant Starch moves though your digestive system, it releases fatty acids that encourage fat burning, especially around your belly.[9]

6. Carbs protect muscle while burning fat!

The right carbs produce a fatty acid that helps you preserve muscle mass—and that stokes your metabolism, thus helping you lose weight faster. When researchers set out to fatten up a bunch of mice, they fed one group of rodents food that was low in Resistant Starch and a second group Resistant Starch-packed food. The mice who were fed the chow that was low in Resistant Starch got fat and flabby—gaining fat and losing muscle mass. Mice that ate the meals high in Resistant Starch preserved their muscle mass, keeping their metabolisms humming along. [10]

7. Carbs blast belly fat!

Carbs help you lose your belly fat faster than other foods, even when the same number of calories are consumed. When scientists fed mice a diet rich in Resistant Starch, it increased the activity of fat-burning enzymes and decreased the activity of fat-storage enzymes. This means that the belly-fat cells were less likely to pick up and store calories as fat. [11]

8. Carbs keep you satisfied!

Carbs keep you satisfied longer than other foods. Here's why: Your brain acts like a computerized fuel gauge that directs you to fill up whenever it notices that its gas tank (your stomach) is empty. It gets these messages from nerves that surround the stomach. It receives messages from various hormones, too. These hormones come from your stomach, your intestines, your pancreas, and your fat cells. Some hormones communicate "empty." Others communicate "full." When many "empty" messages come in at once, the brain turns up those "I'm hungry" signals *and* turns down metabolism. Conversely, when "I'm full" messages come in, appetite decreases and metabolism gets ramped up to fat-burning mode.

Your appetite on carbs

CarbLovers carbs curb hunger better than other types of foods for two reasons. For one thing, they're rich in super-satisfying fiber and Resistant Starch—plus *CarbLovers* carbs are low in calories but high in volume, meaning you get to put way more on your plate. Proof: 3 cups of boiled, diced potatoes have nearly the same amount of calories as 1 cup of shredded Cheddar cheese.

The *CarbLovers* Promise At A Glance

Want to know how eating carbohydrates fills you up on fewer calories, stokes your metabolism, steadies your blood sugar, and lets you eat what you want when you want it? Check out this head-to-toe chart.

Brain You'll be eating foods that help fullness hormones like leptin do their job, turning off appetite and turning up your metabolic furnace.

Mouth *CarbLovers* recipes are high in flavor, but low in calories. They will delight and satisfy your taste buds, allowing you to feel full sooner during a meal.

Stomach Most of the food on this plan is heavy—in a good way. It will weigh down your stomach so you feel full.

Fat cells The Resistant Starch on this plan will trigger fat cells to release their contents so muscle and other cells can burn it for energy.

Bloodstream *CarbLovers* is rich in foods that keep blood sugar levels steady, so you never experience those sudden drops in energy that lead to a stand-in-front-of-the-fridge binge.

Eyes You'll eat frequently on this plan—roughly every few hours. You will also have the opportunity to eat a wide variety of your favorite foods. So no matter how tempting those donuts are in the break room, you'll be able to tell yourself, "I can eat something just as satisfying very soon. I don't need that right now."

Liver Because *CarbLovers* shifts your body into a fat-burning state, your liver will hold onto its stores of glycogen and water. That way, most of the weight you lose early on in this plan will come from fat and not from water.

Gut The high fiber content of the *CarbLovers* plan means that food moves more slowly through your digestive system, causing slow and even rises in blood sugar levels. The Resistant Starch releases fatty acids that turn down appetite, keep blood sugar steady, and turn up fat burning.

Muscles On other diets, you lose muscle. On *CarbLovers,* you'll preserve it, so your metabolism remains stoked.

CarbLovers feeds your body with ultra-satisfying foods—foods that flip on every single fullness trigger in your body. They release fullness hormones in the intestine. They make your cells more sensitive to insulin. They help you get over that initial hump in dieting. By increasing your consumption of filling foods and releasing satiety hormones, *CarbLovers* minimizes the hunger and cravings that makes so many dieters call it quits.

9. Carbs make you feel good—about you!

"Dieters feel so empowered once they lose weight on carbs. For the first time, they are able to lose weight by eating in a balanced manner, without cutting out entire food groups," says Sari Greaves, RD, spokesperson for the American Dietetic Association.

~~~~~~~~~~~~~~~~~

RESISTANT STARCH:
The ULTIMATE
Fat-Burning Carb

You've probably figured out that *The CarbLovers Diet* is going to sneak Resistant Starch into your diet, and you're right! But what the heck is it? Where do you get it? Is it going to bust your budget? And what does it taste like? Relax. Lots of foods you already have in your pantry are loaded with Resistant Starch (see Top Resistant Starch Foods, page 32). And you don't need a lot of Resistant Starch to get dramatic weight-loss results.

Carbohydrate-rich foods (like your old friends bread, potatoes, grains, and fruit) actually contain two types of starch. One is high-glycemic starch. Like sugar, it's absorbed into the bloodstream quickly, raising blood sugar. This also causes a spike in energy. Another is called Resistant Starch, so named because it *resists digestion*. Resistant Starch is neither new nor experimental. As we mentioned earlier, nearly 200 studies have been conducted on Resistant Starch. Most of them are large, multicenter studies published in peer-reviewed medical journals like the *Archives of Internal Medicine*.

These studies show that Resistant Starch is a weight-loss powerhouse because it does not get absorbed into the bloodstream or broken down into glucose. Therefore, it does not raise blood sugar. It travels through your digestive system nearly intact. That's where Resistant Starch triggers the incredible benefits mentioned earlier. It produces fatty acids that promote weight loss by:

- Turning on enzymes that melt fat, especially in the abdominal area.
- Encouraging your liver to switch to a fat-burning state.
- Boosting satiety hormones that make you get and stay full longer. [12]

How Much Resistant Starch Is Enough?

Most people consume only about 4.8 grams of Resistant Starch a day, but researchers believe we need more for optimal health and weight loss. [13] That's why the *CarbLovers* menus include 10 to 15 grams daily of this important fat-burning nutrient, served up in delicious recipes like Chicken Pasta Primavera (page 107) and Coconut French Toast with Raspberry Syrup (page 126).

Resistant Starch is definitely the star on *The CarbLovers Diet,* but it's got a strong supporting cast of foods. This plan doesn't take one "exotic" food and build an entire diet around it—ignoring the fact that you can't live on one food or one food group for the rest of your life. This is about losing weight and keeping it off forever. You'll only be able to do that if all the foods you love are on the menu. Turn to pages 32–33 for a preview of what you'll be eating on *CarbLovers.*

Ask the carb pro
Frances Largeman-Roth, RD

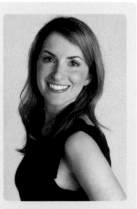

Q. How can I be sure I'm getting enough Resistant Starch?

A. Here's a quick solution: Eat one slightly green banana a day, either in your Banana Shake (page 99) or as a snack. That will guarantee you 12.5 grams of Resistant Starch so you can achieve your weight loss goals without feeling hungry.

"Resistant Starch might sound exotic—but the foods that have it are probably in your kitchen right now! As a bonus, they're affordable, tasty, and easy to prepare."

TOP RESISTANT STARCH FOODS

FOOD	Serving Size	Grams of Resistant Starch per Serving
Banana, green	**1 medium** (7" to 8")	**12.5**
Banana, ripe	1 medium (7" to 8")	4.7
Oatmeal, uncooked/toasted	½ cup	4.6
Beans, white, cooked/canned	½ cup	3.8
Lentils, cooked	½ cup	3.4
Potatoes, cooked and cooled	1 potato, small	3.2
Plantain, cooked	½ cup slices	2.7
Beans, garbanzo, cooked/canned	½ cup	2.1
Pasta, whole-wheat, cooked	1 cup	2.0
Barley, pearl, cooked	½ cup	1.9
Pasta, white, cooked and cooled	1 cup	1.9
Beans, kidney, cooked/canned	½ cup	1.8
Potatoes, boiled (skin & flesh)	1 potato, small	1.8
Rice, brown, cooked	½ cup	1.7
Beans, pinto, cooked/canned	½ cup	1.6
Peas, canned/frozen	½ cup	1.6
Pasta, white, cooked	1 cup	1.5
Beans, black cooked/canned	½ cup	1.5

FOOD	Serving Size	Grams of Resistant Starch per Serving
Millet, cooked	½ cup	1.5
Potatoes, baked (skin & flesh)	1 small	1.4
Bread, pumpernickel	1-ounce slice	1.3
Corn polenta, cooked	½ cup	1.0
Yam, cooked	½ cup cubes	1.0
Potato chips	1 ounce	1.0
Cornflakes	1 cup	0.9
Bread, rye (whole)	1-ounce slice	0.9
Puffed wheat	1¼ cups	0.9
Tortillas, corn	1-ounce, 6" tortilla	0.8
English muffin	1 whole muffin	0.7
Bread, sourdough	1-ounce slice	0.6
Crackers, rye crispbread	2 crispbreads	0.6
Oatmeal, cooked	1 cup	0.5
Bread, Italian	1-ounce slice	0.3
Bread, whole-grain	1-ounce slice	0.3
Corn chips	1 ounce	0.2
Crackers, crispbread (Melba)	½ cup rounds	0.2

"I Lost Weight on *CarbLovers*"

BEFORE

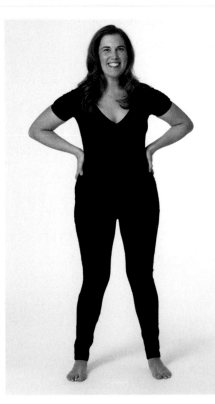

JOY BUTTS

Age: 34

Height: 5'5"

Weight before: 145

Weight after: 136

Pounds lost: 9

Biggest success moment: My out-of-town boyfriend, whom I see every two weeks, jokes that I get smaller every time he sees me.

Biggest challenge: Because of my job, I'm forced to eat out more than most diets allow, so I have to make very conscious choices.

Favorite recipe: Banana Shake (page 99). I can make it before I leave for work, and it kills my sugar cravings.

AFTER

Since I was a teenager, I've tried every diet from Nutrisystem to the Beet Diet. I usually weighed between 130 and 135 pounds. Five years ago, I joined Weight Watchers and got down to 128 pounds. But when I stopped tracking my points, the weight came back on.

Last year my workload increased, which meant late nights and eating anything that wasn't nailed down when I got home at 10 p.m. By July, none of my clothes fit anymore, and I weighed 155 pounds.

I started *CarbLovers* because I hate low-carb diets; I love to run and need fuel for my workouts! I focused on making one *CarbLovers* recipe for breakfast, like the Banana Shake (page 99). The Express Lunch Plate (page 103) seemed like a good fit for my lifestyle, but I was skeptical of how little food it contained. When I tried it, I was shocked that I worked through the entire afternoon without feeling hungry.

When I go out to eat, spotting the whole grains on the menu is easier than I thought. I found a restaurant near my apartment that serves lentil soup with whole-wheat pita bread. I steer my friends to burger joints with whole-grain buns or pizza places with whole-wheat crust.

I always dreaded running while on a diet, but this diet kicked up my energy levels. I've run two marathons before, but I've never felt as strong as I do now. My legs feel strong, and I breathe easily without huffing and puffing! After just two months on *CarbLovers,* I've lost 9 pounds and have more stamina than ever.

Chapter 3

The *CarbLovers* Diet Rules

MOST DIETS FEATURE ONE "star" food or ingredient, and the entire diet is built around it. The trouble is, no one can live on one food or food group without going absolutely nuts! As we mentioned in Chapter 2, while Resistant Starch is definitely the star food in *The CarbLovers Diet,* it has a strong supporting cast. This is a balanced diet, one that includes all the foods you need to look and feel your best. Yes, you'll eat carbs—pasta, bread, potatoes—but you'll also enjoy protein and a little fat, too. And you'll even get wine, chocolate, and other treats. We guarantee you won't waste one minute fixating on what you can't eat. Ready for the new rules that will change the way you eat…for life?

5 Rules of The *CarbLovers* Diet

1. Eat a CarbStar at every meal.

High-in-Resistant-Starch carbs are the cornerstone of this diet. They are your secret to losing weight without hunger or cravings. Resistant Starch is a miracle ingredient found only in carbohydrate foods. *The CarbLovers Diet* maximizes your intake of this fat-flusher by sneaking the top 11 Resistant Starch foods into every meal. We call these Resistant Starch-rich foods **CarbStars!** Each and every one of them contains at least 1 gram of Resistant Starch per serving. Some, like unripe bananas, contain 12 times that much!

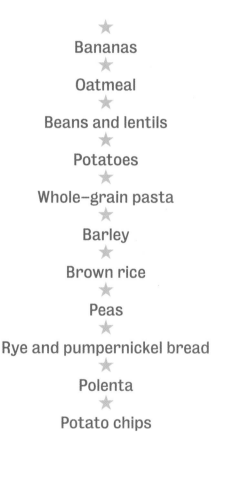

★

Bananas

★

Oatmeal

★

Beans and lentils

★

Potatoes

★

Whole–grain pasta

★

Barley

★

Brown rice

★

Peas

★

Rye and pumpernickel bread

★

Polenta

★

Potato chips

2. Balance your plates.

Depending on where you are in the diet, CarbStars should take up roughly one quarter of your plate. The rest of your meals will be filled with great weight-loss boosters like lean meats and low-fat dairy products, good fats, and fruits and veggies (see the list on pages 254–255). For the first few weeks on *The CarbLovers Diet,* stick to the suggested menus, recipes, and other food options to make sure you get this balancing act just right. Once you reach your goal, you'll find advice in Chapter 10 for building meals on your own, whether you're at home, at work, at a restaurant…even on vacation!

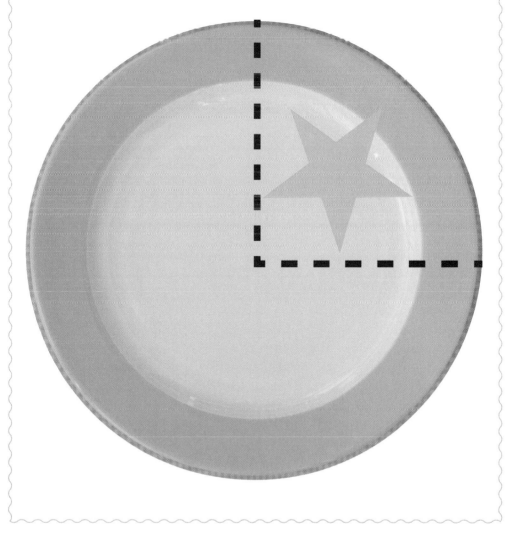

3. Be portion savvy.

Here's the deal on portion control: You can eat the carbs you crave at every meal. That said, you do need to follow our portion advice. The best news, though: We promise you won't feel hungry. You'll discover that the meals on this diet are filling and completely satisfying. (Amazingly, some of our diet testers complained about how often and how much they were eating because they were so used to skipping meals!) The menus and recipes in Chapters 5, 6, and 7 are all carefully calibrated to fill you up—until it's time for your next meal or snack. (That's also true for the frozen dinner and restaurant options we suggest.) On page 256, you'll find a handy chart that helps you create your own versions of *CarbLovers* meals and recipes.

4. Never deprive yourself.

Chocolate desserts, pastas, wine, bread pudding, even potato chips are on *The CarbLovers Diet* menu. Why? When you're forbidden to eat your favorite foods, you end up bingeing on those same foods—and consequently packing on pounds. There's solid research out there that shows this, and yet we continue to follow diets that tell us mostly what we CAN'T eat. I don't know about you, but if I'm told I can't eat pizza, I crave it more than ever, and then when I do break down and have some, I eat about five slices…not just one. On *CarbLovers,* you won't have to give up the one food or beverage that you really love. You can indulge (in moderation) every day.

Your looks on carbs

Switch from a low-carb diet to one that's rich in whole grains, fruits, and veggies, and your skin will start to glow within weeks, says Doris Day, MD, clinical assistant professor of dermatology at New York University. Fruit—especially berries—is a serious beauty booster. It's packed with vitamin C and antioxidants; both improve your skin's elasticity and smooth wrinkles.

5. Build a power pantry.

To succeed with our plan, it's vital that you have a pantry stocked with our CarbStars and other important foods—so you're not tempted to go off the diet. Some of the same fat-burning foods are featured over and over again on this diet. Make sure you have the following within reach at all times:

IN YOUR PANTRY

Almonds, walnuts, other
    nuts and seeds
    (unsalted)
Almond and
    peanut butter (natural)
Baked potato chips
Barley
Brown rice
Canned beans
Coconut, shredded
Cornflakes
Croutons
Dates
Low-fat balsamic
    vinaigrette
Oatmeal (preferably
    rolled or steel cut)
Olive oil
Polenta
Quinoa
Rye crispbread
    crackers
Tortilla chips
Vinegar
Whole-grain bread
Whole-grain pasta

IN YOUR REFRIGERATOR

Berries
Broccoli
Carrots
Low-fat milk
Low-fat cheese
Olives
Pears
Potatoes and sweet potatoes
Salmon
Tortillas
Yogurt, preferably low-fat Greek

IN YOUR FREEZER

Frozen fruit
Frozen meals (see recommendations,
    pages 267–268)
Frozen veggies

ON YOUR COUNTERTOP

Apples
Avocados
Bananas
Pears
Tomatoes

The CarbLovers Diet includes
staples from EVERY food group!

What's on the *CarbLovers* Menu?

Potatoes!

Baked potatoes, sweet potatoes, yams, and even potato chips are on the menu. In addition to **fiber** and **Resistant Starch,** potatoes are a natural source of a proteinase inhibitor, a type of protein which appears to increase levels of satiety hormones and reduce appetite.[1] Potatoes of every stripe are also incredibly filling. One large baked potato, for instance, will run you fewer than 300 calories. Even potato chips are weight-loss friendly, with one serving providing 1 gram of Resistant Starch. They also satisfy your need for crunch, while at the same time providing you with some fiber. If you're going to have a snack chip, then potato chips (preferably baked) are the chips you should reach for.

Beans!

These are true stars of the carb world. Not only are they rich in Resistant Starch, but beans and legumes are also your weight-loss secret weapons because they're one of the few foods that packs both types of fiber—soluble and insoluble. *The CarbLovers Diet* makes sure you get the recommended 25 to 35 grams of fiber every day (see the top fiber-filled foods, page 273). Soluble fiber helps you feel full by absorbing water, and it prevents some of the calories you take in from getting absorbed into your bloodstream. It also slows the absorption of glucose, helping keep your blood sugar levels stable. Insoluble fiber is bulky and fills you up, triggering the feeling of satiety. It also keeps things moving, which prevents bloating. A Brigham Young University study of 252 women found that every 1 gram increase in the amount of fiber consumed correlated with a half a pound of weight loss.[2]

Fruit!

You might have craved other sweets during your last low-carb diet. But lack of fruit probably derailed your weight-loss progress. When Israeli researchers put 322 people on either a low-carb diet, low-fat diet, or a Mediterranean diet, dieters rated fruit—not pasta, not cookies—at the top of their list of longings.[3] "All dieter groups noted fruits as an irresistible food," says Ilana Greenberg, RD, MPH, one of the study's authors. In other words, you can't live without it—and, frankly, there's no reason to try! Certain types of fruit, especially bananas, are rich in Resistant Starch. And other types of fruit are a great source of pectin, a type of soluble fiber found in the rinds and skins of fruit that may block fat storage. In addition to that, fruit is "high volume," and filled with water. This low-calorie density makes it nearly impossible to eat too much fruit. "Fruits and non-starchy vegetables allow you to eat to the point of satisfaction and still lose weight," says Larry Tucker, PhD, a professor at Brigham Young University.

Veggies!

Vegetables such as cucumbers, broccoli, and artichokes are a dieter's best friend. They contain almost no calories (1 cup of raw broccoli has a measly 31 calories!) and are loaded with weight-reducing fiber. So eat up!

Bread, rice, pasta, and whole grains!

The CarbLovers Diet is bringing back tortillas, sandwiches, croutons, and pasta— especially the whole-grain kinds. These foods satisfy our cravings for crunch and chewiness. More important, they are rich in Resistant Starch and fiber, and research shows that people who consume more whole grains tend to weigh less and have less body fat than people who skip them.[4]

Fish!

Cold-water fish like salmon and tuna pack a heart-healthy and slimming fatty acid called **omega-3.** Omega-3s speed weight loss by switching on enzymes that trigger fat-burning in cells. They also help boost mood, which may reduce emotional eating. And omega-3s might improve leptin signaling in the brain, making it turn up fat-burning and turn down appetite. A French study of 27 women determined that adding 3 grams daily of fish oil (the amount in roughly 6 ounces of salmon) reduced body-fat levels by 3.5 percent and abdominal fat by 6 percent.[5] For a list of top omega-3 foods, see page 275.

Nuts and oils!

Most types of nuts and other good-for-you fats, like olive oil, are a rich source of fat-fighting **Monounsaturated Fatty Acids (MUFAs).** One Danish study of 27 men and women found that a diet that included 20 percent of calories from MUFAs measurably sped up 24-hour calorie- and fat-burning after 6 months.[6] Other research shows that MUFAs are especially good at melting tummy fat.[7] High-MUFA foods—namely peanuts, tree nuts, and olive oil—have been shown to keep blood sugar steady and reduce appetite, too. For a list of the top MUFA-rich foods, see page 274.[8]

Meat and dairy!

Steak and macaroni and cheese are on the *CarbLovers* menu for a reason: Both contain **Conjugated Linoleic Acid (CLA),** a fat that is thought to help blood glucose enter body cells so it can be burned for energy and not stored as fat. It's also believed that CLA may help to promote fat burning, especially in muscles, where the bulk of our calorie burning takes place.[9] In an Ohio State University study of 35 women, study participants who took 8 grams of CLA daily lost more weight, especially from fat, compared to women who took a placebo.[10] And a University of Wisconsin study of 23 people who took 4 grams daily of CLA determined that the CLA helped participants burn more fat—even while they were asleep!—than the placebo.[11] Dairy products are also a rich source of calcium, and a University of Tennessee study found that dieters who consumed 1,100 milligrams of calcium daily (upped from 500 milligrams by adding three daily servings of yogurt) lost up to 22 percent more weight and 61 percent more body fat than dieters who had consumed significantly less calcium but had eaten the same number of calories.[12] The reason: Calcium is stored in fat cells, and researchers think that the more calcium a fat cell has, the more fat that cell will release to be burned.

Ask the carb pro

Frances Largeman-Roth, RD

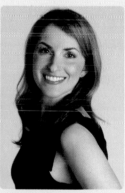

Q. I'm on a budget. Can I still try *CarbLovers*?

A. You bet! To save even more money, try buying your grains—barley, brown rice, and pasta—in bulk. Then store them in airtight containers away from heat and light. This helps them last much longer. Label the container with the name of the grain, the date you purchased it, the correct serving size, and cooking instructions. Plan to use it up within 6 months. To store grains for up to a year, keep them in the fridge or freezer.

"I Lost Weight on *CarbLovers*"

BEFORE

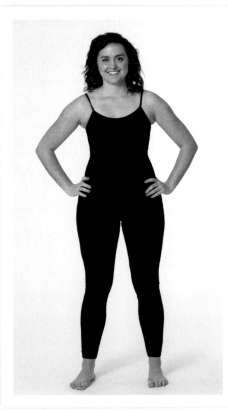

RILEY TANT

Age: 23

Height: 5'8"

Weight before: 167

Weight after: 151

Pounds lost: 16

Biggest success moment: Rocking my favorite black-tweed skirt again. Before, it was SO tight that it rode up when I walked (if I was even able to zip it up that day). Now, I have room to tuck my shirt in!

Biggest challenge: Pizza. It's allowed on *CarbLovers,* but I live above a pizzeria, and the smell is tempting!

Favorite recipe: Chicken Pasta Primavera (page 107). I make it in batches and eat it all week!

AFTER

I started *CarbLovers* for two reasons: I needed a diet that would allow me to cook (even bake!), and I needed to lose the 10-plus pounds I gained during a recent move from Birmingham, Alabama, to New York City. The move was a big adjustment. Take-out food became my new best friend.

CarbLovers **taught me** to substitute healthier carbs for the junk I was eating. It was easy to swap my breakfast cereal for a banana with almond butter and oatmeal, but I was skeptical of other foods, thinking lentils and quinoa would taste like cardboard. Wrong!

After two weeks on *CarbLovers*, I got an unexpected benefit: energy! I could work nine hours a day and then hit the gym for a 4-mile run, five times a week, without feeling exhausted afterward. Even when I started exercising again, I didn't feel hungry on *CarbLovers*. I actually stopped craving sweets after every meal, and my once-a-day chocolate habit became a once-a-week habit with almost no effort.

Friends came to visit midway through my first month on the diet, and I was worried that I would lose control, but I never did. I chose fruit, yogurt, and granola or nuts for breakfast, and then used the portion-control tips on page 39 at lunch and dinner.

I love that *CarbLovers* isn't too strict. The flexibility, in fact, is why my weight is going down, my waist is shrinking, and my energy continues to skyrocket!

Chapter 4

Still
Carbo-Phobic?
Read This!

BY NOW I HOPE all this news about carbs—and how they're going to help you lose weight for life—has you feeling pretty excited. Even if you've just skimmed the previous chapters, you've still discovered that there's a mountain of research—and real-life success stories!—backing up the *CarbLovers* promise: You can lose 15, 35, 100-plus pounds and keep them off, without feeling hungry.

Still, if you're a veteran dieter, you may be a bit wary. Decades of denying yourself potatoes, pasta, bread, and more has you trained to fear carbs. We understand: Carbo-phobia can't be wiped out overnight! All this talk about eating delicious, formerly-forbidden carbs has alarm bells in your head clanging "fattening! fattening! fattening!"

No worries. We're here to help you get your mind as well as your body ready for *CarbLovers*. Read on for eight things you must stop worrying about right now!

8 Carb–Eating Fears to Conquer Right Now

1. Carbs made me heavy in the first place!

The fact is, they didn't. Important research done by big, multicenter studies on thousands of people uncovered this: Slim people eat the most carbs, and the heaviest people eat the least. Still skeptical? Go back to Chapter 2 for details on why carbs did not make you fat—and how *CarbLovers* will make you thin!

2. I'm already eating way too many carbs!

On the contrary, you're probably carb-deficient! The marketers behind fad diets have done a great job convincing people that they are eating too many carbs. In reality, most people eat too few of them—at least the right ones. Consider that for good health and optimal body weight, the country's top nutrition experts recommend you get:

- 25 to 35 grams of fiber (found primarily in carbs) a day. Most people get fewer than 15.
- At least 10 grams of Resistant Starch (found primarily in carbs) a day. Most people get fewer than 4.
- 5 to 9 servings of fruits and vegetables a day. Most people eat fewer than 3.
- 3 servings of whole grains a day. Most people don't even get 1.

3. I'm a carb addict! First, it's a little pasta. Then it's on to bagels, cookies, cake!

Let's back up here. Real food addictions are actually kind of rare: Top experts in the field say they afflict a tiny subset of people, most of whom are severely obese. Even if this describes you, the substances addicts binge on (fatty, sugary, highly processed junk food) bear no resemblance whatsoever to the fresh, nutrient-packed, balanced meals you'll be eating on *The CarbLovers Diet*.

ask the carb pro

Frances Largeman-Roth, RD

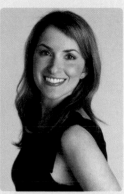

Q. Pasta really freaks me out. Any tips for making friends with this food again?

A. Sure! People mistakenly think "pasta" means piles of starch on a plate. You generally don't sit down to a gigantic mound of brown rice, right? Likewise, pasta should be enjoyed with other flavors and ingredients like fresh herbs, vegetables, lean meats, interesting sauces, and even nuts and beans. Experiment! Go for whole–grain pasta varieties, and try all the cool shapes out there like farfalle (bow–tie), campanelle, fiori, gemelli, and others.

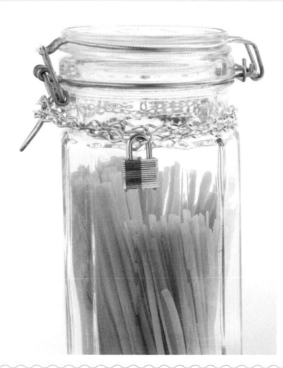

4. So carbs are "in" now. What happens when they're "out" and low-carb is back "in"?

The nutrition science community has always endorsed a carb-rich diet as the best way to stay healthy and slim. As for Resistant Starch? There are hundreds of peer-reviewed, published studies supporting its benefits for health and weight loss (and none suggesting any downsides!). Bottom line: Carbs may be "in" now, but they're honestly here to stay.

5. My favorite celebs don't touch carbs!

You'll make yourself crazy comparing yourself to Hollywood stars, whose careers depend so much on keeping their size 0 figures that some *do* advocate pretty extreme diets, including fasting. *The CarbLovers Diet* was designed for real people who want to get slim and stay that way forever—without starving themselves.

6. Carbs don't fill me up like a good steak!

Whenever you hear people talking about filling foods, they usually mean protein. Yet carbs are the most satisfying foods you can eat (see Chapter 2 for the evidence). And they're the best feel-full bargain around: You can eat double or triple the amount of carbs compared to fat or protein for the same calories. But don't take my word for it—put carbs to the test. Eat them for breakfast (see our list of options on pages 94, 116, and 264) for one week, and try bacon and eggs for another week. I bet you'll find, as I have, that carbs carry you through the day with way more energy and less hunger than other foods.

7. Bread makes me blow up overnight!

What you're talking about here is bloat, not weight gain, and you can't blame carbs for either. It takes an extra 3,500 calories to gain just 1 pound, so unless you devoured more than 3 quarts of full-fat ice cream after dinner, you could not possibly have gained weight overnight. Extra salt is what really makes you blow up, explains Frances Largeman-Roth, RD (my co-author). So if you went to the movies, shared a tub of popcorn with a pal, and then had trouble zipping up your skinny jeans, blame the salt, not the corn! To get right back on track, drink extra water and go easy on packaged and processed foods for a few days.

8. I can't possibly start *CarbLovers* now. My (birthday, vacation, 10th high-school reunion, you fill-in-the-blank) is coming up!

Sure you can. Because right now is the best time to lose weight, and there are so many options for doing it quickly and easily on *The CarbLovers Diet*—without sacrificing your lifestyle. You can have home-cooked family *CarbLovers* meals, at-your-desk lunches, dining-out options…even fast-food choices. Go directly to Chapter 10 for even more details on being a *CarbLover* in any situation.

Your mood on carbs

People feel happier when they include carbs in their diets and crankier when they restrict them, but researchers don't know precisely why this is the case. One theory: Carbs boost the feel-good brain chemical serotonin. Another is that sweet, carb-rich foods elevate mood-boosting opiates in the brain, triggering pleasurable sensations.

"I Lost Weight on *CarbLovers*"

BEFORE

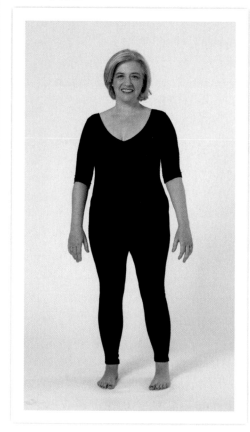

ROSEMARY SHMAVONIAN

Age: 48

Height: 5'4"

Weight before: 165

Weight after: 155

Pounds lost: 10

Biggest success moment: I have a floral dress that my husband bought me years ago. It barely fit when I got it, but I'm wearing it to a wedding this spring. And it looks great!

Biggest challenge: Finding the time to grocery shop. But once I stocked my cabinets with barley, quinoa, and beans, I was set for months!

Favorite recipe: White Bean Salsa & Chips (page 199). It tastes like no diet food I've ever had!

AFTER

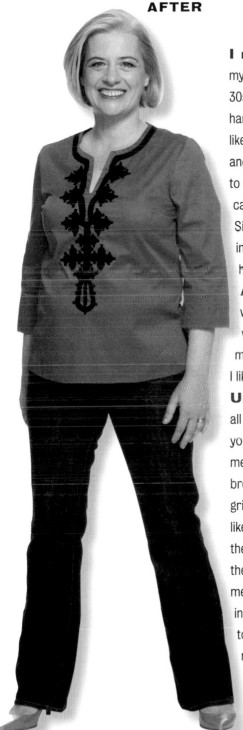

I never battled with my weight until after my two pregnancies. I had my boys in my late 30s, and losing 40 pounds post-pregnancy was harder than I thought! I've tried low-carb diets like South Beach before, but I was hungry, cranky, and the scale didn't move. *CarbLovers* appealed to me because I needed a diet that fit into our carb-eating family's lifestyle and not just mine. Since my husband has high cholesterol, the fiber in these recipes seemed like a healthy choice for him, too.

At first my weight loss was slow. But by week three, I had dropped 7 pounds. The weight just fell off my troublesome areas, like my belly and hips. Even if the scale didn't move, I liked the way my body was changing shape.

Unlike other diets, this one emphasizes all the foods you *can* eat, instead of all the foods you can't. It's been surprisingly easy to craft meals, even when I've been traveling. At a recent breakfast buffet I went for *CarbLovers*-approved grits, smoked fish, and fruit. It was delicious! I felt like I wasn't restricting food, but substituting all the junk I'd been eating with healther foods. And there's nothing you absolutely can't have, which means I can stick with it! Incorporating *CarbLovers* ingredients like barley and quinoa into my day-to-day life has helped me drop 10 pounds in two months. But more important, it's setting up healthy habits for my family.

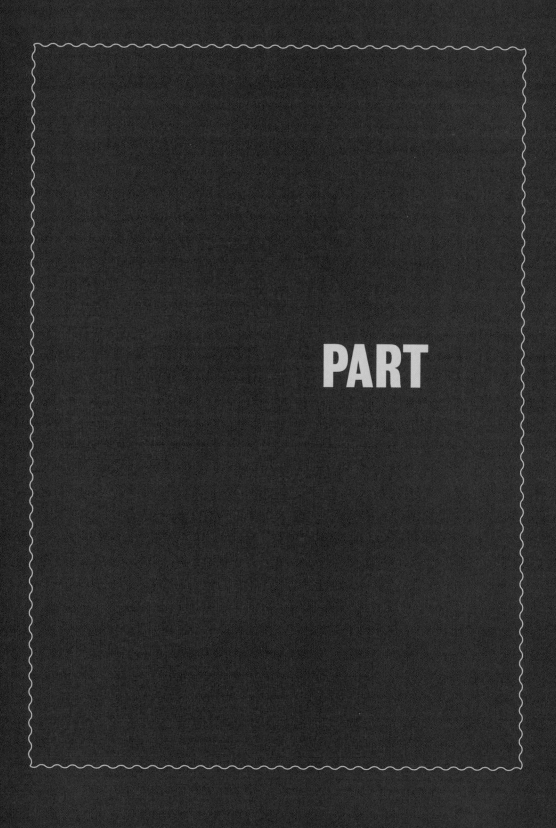

PART

The CarbLovers Plan

Chapter 5

PHASE 1:
The 7-Day *CarbLovers* Kickstart Plan

THE NEXT SEVEN DAYS WILL CHANGE YOUR LIFE FOREVER. They make up the first phase of The *CarbLovers* Diet Plan. It is designed to help you lose up to 6 pounds with minimal effort. What you do for the next week will also set the stage for even bigger achievements (including truly dramatic weight loss!) in Phase 2 of *CarbLovers*. Following this plan will improve your life in four ways you never dreamed possible:

1. Your longing for real food and feelings of deprivation will end forever because you'll be nourished with the foods your body has been hungry for…maybe even since your childhood.

2. You'll feel more energized and in control than you have in years because you won't be skipping meals.

3. You'll relax <u>and</u> enjoy eating carbs again because you'll be losing weight on carb-rich foods.

4. You'll feel a whole lot happier because you'll finally be eating the carbs your body and brain craves—and you'll also be losing weight.

Favorite recipes: The sharp Cheddar & Egg on Rye *, and the Cherry Ginger Scones * — the oatmeal was tasty... must remember to bring snack on Monday and drink more water!

"Write down what you eat! Keeping a food diary is one of the best predictors of weight loss."

IN THIS CHAPTER, you'll learn everything you need to drop real weight, real fast—without ever going hungry! We're going to give you seven days' worth of meals and snacks. You'll be able to enjoy delicious, easy recipes for those times when you want to cook and suggestions for prepared, grab-and-go meals for when you don't. You'll be able to stick to *CarbLovers* on the road, at the office, in a restaurant, at a party—pretty much wherever you find yourself this week. Our 7-Day *CarbLovers* Kickstart Meal Plan starts on page 66 and includes advice from experts and real-life dieters to help you stay the course and lose weight.

The *CarbLovers* Kickstart Plan eases you into *CarbLovers* eating gently, so you'll never be tempted to stray. If you're still nervous about diving into a diet that puts carbs back on the plate, these three hallmarks of the plan will reassure you:

1. The 7-Day *CarbLovers* Kickstart Plan = 1,200 calories a day.

For the next seven days, you can simply follow the menu we've created—or you can mix and match the meals any way you choose. Either way, you'll lose that first 6 pounds or so. By the way, we understand if you're a little skeptical about the whole "carbs are my weight-loss friend" concept. Just know that whether you follow the menu to the letter or mix and match the meal choices, the 1,200 daily calories you get lead to only one outcome: rapid weight loss.

2. *CarbLovers* Kickstart was tested on real people.

Before we began to work on these menus, we recruited women of different ages, shapes, and lifestyles to test our plan. Some were career-focused women, others were stay-at-home moms. Some had a lot of weight to lose, while others only wanted to drop 10 pounds. But they did have one important thing in common: They all lost big on The 7-Day *CarbLovers* Kickstart Plan—from 3 pounds to a whopping 6 pounds in seven days! Most important, they gave us no-holds-barred feedback on what worked best for them. For example, some wanted foods they could share with their families, while others were eager for fast-food options. Some loved salads, while others were more interested in heartier fare. A couple of them started exercising on the diet and wanted a bit more food. Others were so satisfied that they actually wanted to eat less. We listened. With their input, we created a plan that not only guarantees weight loss, but is also flexible enough to work with any lifestyle. And the best news: All of our testers said they felt satisfied and filled with energy while they lost weight.

3. Anyone can stick to this plan.

The dietitians who designed these menus and recipes went the extra mile to keep them as simple as possible. The day-by-day *CarbLovers* Kickstart Meal Plan eliminates guesswork, and even if you don't cook, you can easily follow along: There are as many on-the-go, no-cook choices as there are recipes.

~~~~~~~~~~

THE 7-DAY *CARBLOVERS* KICKSTART RULES
(Read this before you start!)

◼ Don't cut out the carbs!

This plan puts you in control, but please—don't "adapt" it by cutting carbs. These foods were carefully designed to satisfy your cravings for brain- and body-nourishing nutrients that keep you feeling full. Cutting carbs will only trigger binges that keep you from your weight-loss goal.

◼ Do write down what you eat.

Keeping a food diary will help you lose weight and train you to incorporate carbs into your life again. University of Pittsburgh researchers found that dieters who consistently jotted down what they ate (and when) lost weight more quickly than dieters who didn't.[1] Researchers also found that keeping a food diary helped dieters follow their plans without backsliding or cheating, even after a full year.[2]

Keep your food diary either on paper or digitally (try the notes function on your cell phone). As you jot down what you eat, place stars next to "Foods that are high in Resistant Starch" (see page 272 for a list), "Foods that boost metabolism" (see pages 270–271 for lists of foods that are rich in MUFAs, omega-3s, and more), and "Foods that are high in fiber." This way, you'll quickly commit to memory the foods that you should be eating going forward.

◼ Don't lean on artificial sweeteners.

Here's why I want you to ban the fake stuff on this diet: Studies suggest that artificial sweeteners (especially in diet sodas) don't promote weight loss and may even increase your cravings for sugary foods—thus helping you pack on pounds. Fake sweeteners are up to 600 times sweeter than sugar, but they aren't even real carbs! Consuming them every day numbs your taste buds to the natural sweetness of good-for-you carbs like bananas, berries, and other fresh fruit.

Prepare the same meals often.

Getting used to *CarbLovers* recipes serves a dual purpose. First, it's convenient. The more often you make something, the easier it is for you to re-create. All of the *CarbLovers* Kickstart lunch and dinner options can be used during the 21-Day *CarbLovers* Immersion Plan and beyond, so it makes sense to get to know them. Eventually, you won't even need this book. You'll be able to shop for the right ingredients and create the meals on your own.

Second, we want you to be able to take this plan anywhere. Say you're on *CarbLovers* and you have to visit family across the country. If you're familiar with shopping for and assembling *CarbLovers* meals, you can stick to your diet in anyone's kitchen without a problem. They'll probably become converts to the diet just by trying your meals for a day or two!

Eat one snack a day.

Snacking is important on this plan because having snacks prevents between-meal bingeing. But when you snack is up to you. If you're not sure when to have your snack, try it two to three hours after lunch. If you're a night owl, go ahead and

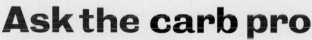

Ask the carb pro

Frances Largeman-Roth, RD

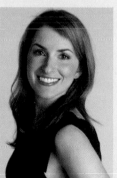

Q. Can I eat breakfast for dinner— and vice versa—on *CarbLovers?*

A. Yes. Some people feel safer and more in control when they eat the same thing every day—even if it's a shake for dinner or pasta for breakfast! If that describes you, then go for it. It may make it easier for you to stick to the plan.

have your mini-treat an hour or two after dinner. *Note:* It's fine to snack after breakfast, but most of our diet testers found that the longer they waited to eat their snack, the easier it was to stick to the diet.

▣ Don't skip meals.

The 7-Day *CarbLovers* Kickstart Plan purposely includes breakfast, lunch, dinner, and one snack. While lots of dieters take pride in their meal-skipping abilities, we don't want you to skip—EVER! You must stick to this pattern in order to maintain your blood sugar levels (and thus your energy) and keep hunger at bay. Skipping just one meal will make you feel tired and stressed—and more likely to pig out later.

▣ Keep trigger foods out of the house.

By the end of the 21-Day *CarbLovers* Immersion Plan in Chapter 6, you'll be able to consume carbs with confidence. But you're not there yet. So keep foods that make you act out-of-control crazy (mine is chocolate-chip cookie dough) out of the house, where they're less likely to make you to lose your self-control.

▣ Don't drink liquid calories.

For the next seven days, you can drink water, coffee, and tea (black, green, or herbal, without sweeteners, but with up to 2 teaspoons of low-fat milk), and my secret Fat-Flushing Cocktail (below). The Fat-Flushing Cocktail includes powerful metabolism-boosting ingredients that will help speed you to your goal. Skip fruit juice, alcoholic, and carbonated beverages (even diet sodas or sparkling water), which make you look and feel bloated.

Fat-Flushing Cocktail

Ellen Kunes, Editor in Chief, *Health* magazine

Shhh...this drink is my secret, an all-natural diet aid that tastes great. The tea may help you burn off an extra 80 calories a day, and the citrus gives it a naturally sweet punch. Whether you want to share it is up to you!

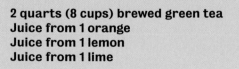

2 quarts (8 cups) brewed green tea
Juice from 1 orange
Juice from 1 lemon
Juice from 1 lime

Mix all ingredients together in one large pitcher. Serve hot or iced; store it in the fridge for up to 3 days.

PHASE 1:
THE 7-DAY *CARBLOVERS* KICKSTART MEAL PLAN

This plan makes eating the *CarbLovers* way a no-brainer. We've included at-a-glance meals, and even grab-and-go, restaurant, and frozen options for dieters who don't have time to cook! Where there's room, we've written out the recipe in the menus—even when it appears again in Chapter 7—so you don't have to flip pages. Feel free to mix and match any course in any menu, and don't even think about skipping meals!

The 7-Day Checklist

☐ **Sit down to every meal:** Grabbing something and eating it over the sink sets you up for overeating. It doesn't give you a chance to be mindful about your food, and you're less likely to pay attention to the serving size. Sit down and enjoy!

☐ **Stay hydrated:** Sometimes we mistake thirst for hunger, so hydrate! Drink eight (8-ounce) glasses of water each day.

☐ **Tell the world you're on a diet:** OK, maybe not everyone, but telling a few close friends will help keep you honest and motivated.

☐ **Ditch distractions:** TV, music, and even dinner companions can cause you to overeat.

☐ **Slow down:** Try to relax and slow down while you eat. You'll enjoy your food more and will eat less!

☐ **Nix family-style:** Instead of putting out all of the *CarbLovers* recipe you cooked, portion out your plate and enjoy that amount. You'll eat less without feeling deprived.

☐ **Raid Grandma's china cabinet:** The dinner plates we use today are far bigger than they used to be. Pick up smaller ones from Grandma or find some at a garage sale. Or try using your salad plate instead of your dinner plate. It will feel like you have a lot more food on your plate!

MONDAY (DAY 1)

Breakfast
Banana Shake (page 99): Blend 1 banana, 1½ cups 1% low-fat milk, 2 teaspoons honey, and ½ cup ice.
or
Kashi TLC Chewy Granola Bar plus 1 banana

Lunch
Chicken Pita Sandwich (page 102): 1 cup baby spinach, ½ cup sliced bell pepper, and 4 ounces cooked skinless, boneless chicken strips, tossed with 2 tablespoons low-fat Italian vinaigrette, and stuffed into 1 (6-inch) whole-grain pita (halved).
or
Tuna or chicken salad kits (brands such as StarKist or Bumble Bee) plus pear (1 medium) plus string cheese (1)

Dinner
Skillet Salmon & Parmesan Potatoes (page 112)
or
Amy's Black Bean Vegetable Enchilada

Snack
Greek yogurt (¾ cup, plain low-fat) plus honey (2 teaspoons) plus rolled oats (2 tablespoons, uncooked or toasted)

TUESDAY (DAY 2)

Breakfast
Banana-Nut Oatmeal (page 96)
or
1 banana plus 1 teaspoon peanut or almond butter

Lunch
Express Lunch Plate (page 103):
1 large hard-cooked egg, 1 ounce cheddar cheese, and 1 sliced apple, served with 3 rye crispbread crackers.
or
Tuna or chicken salad kits (brands such as StarKist or Bumble Bee) plus pear (1 medium) plus 1 string cheese

Dinner
Shrimp Stir-Fry with Ginger (page 111)
or
Boca veggie burger with 1 toasted whole-grain bun and 1 teaspoon mustard plus 1 medium apple

Snack
White Bean & Herb Hummus with Crudités (page 115): ¼ cup canned white beans (rinsed and drained) mashed with 2 teaspoons olive oil, 1 tablespoon chopped chives, and 1 tablespoon lemon juice. Serve dip with ½ cup sliced raw vegetables.

WEDNESDAY (DAY 3)

Breakfast
Banana Shake Plus (page 99):
Blend 1 banana, 1½ cups 1% low-fat milk, 2 teaspoons honey, ½ cup ice, and 2 tablespoons ground flaxseed.

Lunch
Big Chopped Salad (page 100)
or
Tuna or chicken salad kits (brands such as StarKist or Bumble Bee) plus pear (1 medium) plus 1 string cheese

Dinner
Black Bean Tacos (page 104)
or
2 cups (1 can) Progresso High Fiber Homestyle Minestrone with 3 rye crispbread crackers

Snack
Salsa (2 tablespoons) plus canned black beans (2 tablespoons, rinsed and drained), served with corn tortilla chips (8)

THURSDAY (DAY 4)

Breakfast
Banana-Berry Shake (page 99):
Blend 1 banana, 1½ cups 1% low-fat
milk, 2 teaspoons honey, ½ cup ice,
and ¼ cup berries.

or

Kashi TLC Chewy Granola Bar
plus 1 banana

Lunch
Chicken Pita Sandwich (page 102):
1 cup baby spinach, ½ cup sliced
bell pepper, and 4 ounces cooked
skinless, boneless chicken strips,
tossed with 2 tablespoons low-fat
Italian vinaigrette, and stuffed into
1 (6-inch) whole-grain pita (halved).

or

Boca veggie burger with 1 toasted
whole-grain bun and 1 teaspoon
mustard plus 1 medium apple

Dinner
Chicken Pasta Primavera (page
107)

or

Amy's Black Bean Vegetable Enchilada

Snack
Almond butter (2 teaspoons) with rye
crispbread crackers (2)

FRIDAY (DAY 5)

Breakfast
Banana & Almond Butter Toast
(page 95): 1 toasted slice of rye bread
topped with 1 tablespoon almond
butter and 1 sliced banana.

or

½ cup Fiber One cereal with ½ cup
1% low-fat milk and ½ sliced banana

Lunch
Express Lunch Plate (page 103):
1 large hard-cooked egg, 1 ounce
cheddar cheese, and 1 sliced apple,
served with 3 rye crispbread crackers.

or

Amy's Black Bean Vegetable Enchilada

Dinner
Grilled Burger & 3-Bean Salad
(page 108)

or

Lean Cuisine Salmon with Basil plus
2 cups salad greens with low-fat
vinaigrette

Snack
Trail Mix (page 114):
cornflakes (½ cup) plus sliced
almonds (2 tablespoons) plus dried
cherries (2 tablespoons).

SATURDAY (DAY 6)

Breakfast
Banana-Cocoa Shake (page 99):
Blend 1 banana, 1½ cups 1% low-fat
milk, 2 teaspoons honey, ½ cup ice,
and 1 tablespoon unsweetened cocoa.
or
Kashi TLC Chewy Granola Bar
plus 1 banana

Lunch
Big Chopped Salad (page 100)
or
2 cups (1 can) Progresso High Fiber
Homestyle Minestrone with 3 rye
crispbread crackers

Dinner
Boca veggie burger with 1 toasted
whole-grain bun and 1 teaspoon
mustard plus 1 medium apple
or
2 cups (1 can) Progresso High Fiber
Homestyle Minestrone with 3 rye
crispbread crackers

Snack
Greek yogurt (¾ cup, plain low-fat)
plus honey (2 teaspoons) plus rolled
oats (2 tablespoons, uncooked or
toasted)

SUNDAY (DAY 7)

Breakfast
Banana & Almond Butter Toast
(page 95): 1 toasted slice of rye bread
topped with 1 tablespoon almond
butter and 1 sliced banana.
or
½ cup Fiber One cereal with ½ cup
1% low-fat milk and ½ sliced banana

Lunch
Express Lunch Plate (page 103):
1 large hard-cooked egg, 1 ounce
cheddar cheese, and 1 sliced apple,
served with 3 rye crispbread crackers.
or
Lean Cuisine Salmon with Basil plus
2 cups salad greens with low-fat
vinaigrette

Dinner
**Skillet Salmon & Parmesan
Potatoes** (page 112)
or
Boca veggie burger with 1 toasted
whole-grain bun and 1 teaspoon
mustard plus 1 medium apple

Snack
Baked potato chips (24 chips, about
1 ounce)

"I Lost Weight on CarbLovers"

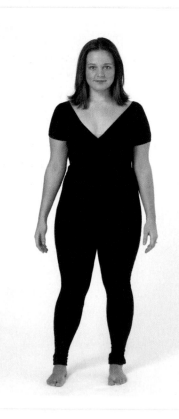

CAITLIN GRAMS

Age: 24

Height: 5'3"

Weight before: 154

Weight after: 145

Pounds lost: 9

Biggest success moment: Fitting into a pair of skinny jeans I'd been eyeing.

Biggest challenge: Facing my fear of rice, pasta, and bread! *CarbLovers* really helped me overcome my carbo-phobia!

Favorite recipe: Dark Chocolate & Oat Clusters (page 213). Two of these clusters completely satisfy my sweet tooth, and my husband LOVES them.

AFTER

It's ironic and eye-opening that I had success on *The CarbLovers Diet* because I was someone who always banned rice, passed on the bread basket, and limited pasta, which was difficult when I married into an Italian family!

I've been overweight most of my life. Though I've always been a runner, I was never good at portion control. About three years ago, I hit my heaviest weight, 185 pounds. I tried other diets, but they seemed so boring and gimmicky after awhile.

***CarbLovers* seemed different** but I was a little afraid I would be hungry, especially during Phase 1. But after two or three days of eating the whole grains, I realized I wasn't starving at all. I'm not a huge lunch person, but this diet forced me to eat it. I always thought salads were dull, but the chopped salad on this diet combined garbanzo beans and purple cabbage— two things I never would have added to my greens!

In the past I felt like I always needed more sleep, but on *CarbLovers* I slept the same amount and had more energy throughout the day. My fitness goal was to run two 6-mile loops in Central Park. The foods I ate on *CarbLovers* fueled my runs and gave me the energy to achieve my goal!

In two months, I've lost 9 pounds and feel completely in control of my eating habits.

Chapter 6

PHASE 2:
The 21-Day *CarbLovers* Immersion Plan

BY NOW YOU'RE PROBABLY AT LEAST 6 POUNDS LIGHTER, and you're enjoying a new, healthier relationship with yummy foods you haven't eaten in a long time. Best of all, you're bursting with energy! It's time to take your slimmed-down self and get ready for the next phase of *CarbLovers* because the best is yet to come. In Phase 2 of *The CarbLovers Diet*, called The 21-Day *CarbLovers* Immersion Plan, you'll be adding even more favorite foods (think steak and potato dinners, French toast for breakfast, even the occasional chocolate treat). Portion sizes will increase, and you'll be able to order from the menu at your favorite restaurants.

You'll eat all this, and you'll still lose another 6 pounds—or even more. On The 21-Day *CarbLovers* Immersion Plan, you actually get to eat 1,600 calories a day (up from the 1,200 calories you had on The 7-Day *CarbLovers* Kickstart Plan). Losing weight gets even easier during this part of *CarbLovers* because The 21-Day *CarbLovers* Immersion Plan is designed to fit in perfectly with your unique lifestyle. Before you dive into the menu and meal plan, check out how to make it work best for you.

You have two great options here:

1. You can build your own customized daily menus by mixing and matching meal choices from our *CarbLovers* Recipe Collection (starting on page 93) and from more than 100 packaged, fast-food, and/or restaurant meals. All of these amazing options start on page 264.

2. Or for those of you who prefer more guidance, we've created a 21-day meal plan you'll absolutely love, starting on page 78. These menus were developed by our dietitians and tested on a group of incredibly busy women. They told us this plan was easy to follow—and that not having to create their own menus every day made losing weight 100 percent stress-free.

Most important: **All *CarbLovers* meals are interchangeable,** and any combination will help you lose weight. Eat the same thing for breakfast every day, if that keeps it easy for you—or eat one of our dinners for lunch or a favorite breakfast for dinner, if you feel like it. It all adds up to fat-burning and weight loss!

Your goals for the next three weeks are to:

Lose about 2 pounds each week. By the end of the *CarbLovers* Kickstart and *CarbLovers* Immersion Phases, most dieters say they've lost a total of at least 12 pounds—without feeling hungry!

Relax and enjoy eating carbs! You've now got proof that you can eat bread, rice, pasta, and more without fear.

Know how to spot appetite-suppressors like fiber, Resistant Starch, and MUFAs in prepared foods—and make smart choices if you stray from the plan.

■ **Feel confident** about converting *CarbLovers* from a diet to a way of life. At the end of three weeks, preparing *CarbLovers* meals will become second nature.

How is The 21-Day *CarbLovers* Immersion Plan different from the Kickstart Plan?

■ You get to eat more!

You'll get larger portions than you did during The 7-Day *CarbLovers* Kickstart Plan. Many of our test dieters told us that they were so satisfied with these meals that they could not finish what was on their plates. We actually had to coach them to eat their snacks!

■ You get lots of choices!

This plan includes super-satisfying meals, decadent treats, and fast food and/or restaurant options that appeal to every palate. You won't feel as if you are on a diet so you'll have a much easier time sticking with the plan.

■ You get plenty of treats!

Dessert! Wine! Cappuccino! Every day, you get to choose two snacks (compared to one on The 7-Day *CarbLovers* Kickstart Plan), and one of these snacks can be an indulgence chosen from the list provided on page 116. From ice cream and chocolate-covered bananas to sweet potato pudding, you won't believe what you can enjoy and still lose weight!

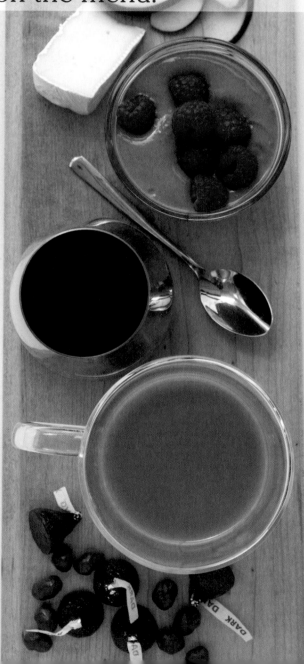

This is diet food? You bet. On *CarbLovers*, treats are on the menu!

PHASE 2:
THE 21-DAY *CARBLOVERS* IMMERSION MEAL PLAN

TO GET YOU STARTED on the next phase of *CarbLovers*, here are three weeks of menu suggestions. We've included at-a-glance meals and even grab-and-go, restaurant, and frozen options for dieters who don't have time to cook. (There are lots more of those in Chapter 11, too.) Where there's room, we've written out the recipe in the menus—even when it appears again in Chapter 7—so you don't have to flip pages if you're in a hurry. Feel free to mix and match any meal in any menu!

21-Day Checklist

■ **Keep track of snacks:** If you run or walk more than 5 miles a day and/or you start to feel really hungry or tired, go ahead and double the size of one of your snacks. If you're not losing weight at all, cut one out.

■ **When you feel full, stop eating!** Don't feel like you should clean your plate. The suggested portions in the menu options and recipes are just that—suggestions. Many of our test dieters said that portions were sometimes too big for them. If you feel too full after meals, scale back.

■ **Mix and match:** Incorporate your favorite menu options from The 7-Day *CarbLovers* Kickstart Plan into The 21-Day *CarbLovers* Immersion Plan. All of the meal options from Phase 1 of our diet will also work during Phase 2.

MONDAY (DAY 1)

Breakfast
Breakfast Barley with Banana & Sunflower Seeds (page 119): Mix ⅓ cup quick-cooking barley with ⅔ cup water and microwave for 6 minutes. Let stand for 2 minutes, then top with 1 teaspoon honey, 1 sliced banana, and 1 tablespoon sunflower seeds.
or
Panera Strawberry Granola Parfait

Lunch
Ham, Sliced Pear & Swiss Sandwich (page 146)
or
6" Subway Veggie Delite Sandwich on 9-grain wheat bread

Dinner
Roasted Pork Tenderloin with Apricot-Barley Pilaf (page 186)
or
Healthy Choice Oven Roasted Chicken

Snack #1
Antipasto Platter (page 209): 12 canned black olives (drained), ½ cup marinated artichoke hearts (drained), and ½ red bell pepper (sliced).

Snack #2
1 ounce dark chocolate-covered cherries (about 3)

TUESDAY (DAY 2)

Breakfast
Banana Yogurt Parfait with Maple Oat Topping (page 118)
or
Au Bon Pain Apple Cinnamon Oatmeal (12 ounces, medium)

Lunch
Tuscan Barley Salad (page 165)
or
Fazoli's Grilled Chicken Artichoke Salad

Dinner
Sirloin Salad with Blue Cheese Dressing & Sweet Potato Fries (page 181)
or
Healthy Choice Café Steamers Chicken Pesto Classico

Snack #1
Pistachio & Dried Cherry Crostini (page 209): 2 tablespoons low-fat cottage cheese mixed with 1 teaspoon honey, 2 teaspoons chopped pistachios, and 2 teaspoons chopped dried cherries, served on top of 2 rye crispbread crackers.

Snack #2
1 Reese's Peanut Butter Cup (half of a 1.5-ounce package)

WEDNESDAY (DAY 3)

Breakfast
Tomato & Mozzarella Melt (page 136)
or
Starbucks Apple Bran Muffin with Omega-3s & 7g Fiber

Lunch
Big Chopped Salad (page 100)
or
Così Hummus & Veggie Sandwich

Dinner
Barley Risotto Primavera (page 166)
or
Marie Callender's Honey Roasted Turkey

Snack #1
Brie and apple slices (page 209): 1 small sliced apple with 1 ounce Brie.

Snack #2
One glass of red wine (5 ounces)

THURSDAY (DAY 4)

Breakfast
Broccoli & Feta Omelet with Toast
(page 122)
or
Dunkin' Donuts Ham, Egg White &
Cheese on Wheat English Muffin

Lunch
Pesto Turkey Club (page 158)
and 1 apple
or
Jamba Juice Chimichurri Chicken
Wrap without sauce
or
Any 6" Subway Sandwich on 9-grain
wheat bread

Dinner
**Fish Tacos with Sesame-Ginger
Slaw** (page 172)
or
Kashi Lemongrass Coconut Chicken

Snack #1
Fig & Flax Yogurt (page 209): Mix ½
cup low-fat plain Greek yogurt with
1 teaspoon honey, 3 dried, chopped
figs, and 1 teaspoon ground flaxseeds.

Snack #2
Grande (16 ounce) cappuccino,
regular or decaf, with 2% low-fat milk

FRIDAY (DAY 5)

Breakfast
Sharp Cheddar & Egg on Rye
(page 134)
or
Jamba Juice Coldbuster (16 ounces)

Lunch
**Roast Beef Sandwich with
Horseradish Aioli** (page 161):
serve with 1 cup sliced cucumbers
and 1 tablespoon light Italian dressing.
or
P.F. Chang's Buddha's Feast steamed
with a side of brown rice

Dinner
**Mediterranean Seafood Grill
with Skordalia** (page 175)
or
Kashi Black Bean Mango Pilaf

Snack #1
**Greek Yogurt with Orange
Marmalade & Walnuts** (page 209):
½ cup low-fat plain Greek yogurt
mixed with 2 teaspoons 100% fruit
orange marmalade and 1 tablespoon
chopped walnuts

Snack #2
Chocolate-Orange Spoonbread
(page 214)

SATURDAY (DAY 6)

Breakfast
Cherry-Ginger Scones (page 125)
or
Jimmy Dean D-lights Turkey Bacon
Bowl

Lunch
Black Bean & Zucchini
Quesadillas (page 141)
or
Wendy's Small Chili with Side Salad

Dinner
Baked Two-Cheese Penne with
Roasted Red Pepper Sauce
(page 192)
or
Kashi Ranchero Beans

Snack #1
Honey-Curried Yogurt Dip with
Carrots & Broccoli (page 209): Mix
½ cup low-fat plain Greek yogurt with
1 teaspoon honey, ¼ teaspoon curry
powder, and ⅛ teaspoon salt. Serve
with ½ cup each of baby carrots and
broccoli florets.

Snack #2
Dark Chocolate & Oat Clusters
(page 213)

SUNDAY (DAY 7)

Breakfast
Potato-Crusted Spinach Quiche
(page 133)
or
Aunt Jemima Sausage & Egg Scramble

Lunch
Arugula Salad with Lemon Dijon
Dressing (page 138)
or
6" Subway Veggie Delite Sandwich on
9-grain wheat bread

Dinner
Thai Peanut Noodles (page 190)
or
Wendy's Sour Cream & Chives Potato

Snack #1
Hummus with Feta & Dill
(page 209): Top 4 tablespoons
original hummus (store-bought tub)
with 1 tablespoon feta cheese and
⅛ teaspoon dried dill. Serve with
1 cup sliced cucumber.

Snack #2
5 Hershey's Special Dark Kisses

21-Day Checklist (continued)

■ **Prevent plateaus:** If your weight-loss stalls during The 21-Day *CarbLovers* Immersion Plan, you can go back to The 7-Day *CarbLovers* Kickstart Plan to jump-start your diet again. You *will* lose all the weight you want on *CarbLovers;* it just might take you a bit longer.

■ **Don't skip meals or snacks in an attempt to speed up your pounds-off results:** Doing so will backfire by triggering cravings. If you really think you're eating too much food, shrink your portions slightly. But whatever you do, don't skip meals!

■ **Go bananas:** These menus have been created to ensure you consume at least 10 grams of Resistant Starch a day. Bananas are a big part of that secret formula because they contain more Resistant Starch than any other single food (4.7 grams, and even more for a green one!). But if you are simply tired of bananas (or out of them), eat any medium-sized piece of fruit or 1 cup of berries.

MONDAY (DAY 8)

Breakfast
Oatmeal with Dried Plum & Banana Compote (page 128)
or
Subway Egg & Cheese Sandwich on 9-grain bread with egg white

Lunch
Middle Eastern Rice Salad (page 153)
or
Amy's Spinach Feta in a Pocket Sandwich

Dinner
Spanish-Style Shrimp with Yellow Rice (page 182)
or
Wendy's Southwest Taco Salad

Snack #1
Salmon & Cream Cheese Bites (page 209): Spread 2 teaspoons low-fat cream cheese on 1 slice toasted pumpernickel bread. Top with ½ ounce smoked salmon and 2 teaspoons chopped chives.

Snack #2
10 Goobers chocolate-covered peanuts

TUESDAY (DAY 9)

Breakfast
Cornflakes, Low-Fat Milk & Berries (page 127): 2 cups cornflakes served with 1 cup low-fat milk and topped with 1 cup fresh or thawed frozen berries.
or
Smart Ones Stuffed Breakfast Sandwich plus 1 banana

Lunch
Smoked Salmon & Avocado Hand Rolls (page 162)
or
Amy's Bean & Rice Burrito

Dinner
Pan-Seared Scallops with Southwestern Rice Salad (page 178)
or
6" Subway Oven-Roasted Chicken Sandwich on 9-grain wheat bread

Snack #1
Cheddar & Apple Melt (page 208): Place 1 tablespoon shredded cheddar cheese and 1 small thinly-sliced apple in 1 corn tortilla. Microwave for 30 seconds until cheese is bubbling.

Snack #2
1 Skinny Cow ice-cream cone

WEDNESDAY (DAY 10)

Breakfast
Apple & Almond Muesli (page 117): Combine ½ cup rolled oats with ½ cup low-fat milk, and let sit for 5 to 10 minutes. Stir in 1 chopped apple, 2 tablespoons sliced almonds, and 2 teaspoons honey.
or
2 Eggo Nutri-Grain Waffles plus 1 banana

Lunch
Express Lunch Plate (page 103): 1 hard boiled egg, 1 ounce cheddar cheese, and 1 sliced apple served with 3 rye crispbread crackers.
or
Lean Cuisine Sun-Dried Tomato Pesto Chicken

Dinner
Caribbean Mahi Mahi with Banana Chutney (page 171)
or
Jamba Juice Chimichurri Chicken Wrap without sauce

Snack #1
Chili-Spiked Pita Chips (page 202)

Snack #2
Banana Ice Cream (page 210)

THURSDAY (DAY 11)

Breakfast
Zucchini & Potato Scramble with Bacon (page 137)
or
Two Vita Tops (Banana Nut) plus 1 banana

Lunch
Moroccan Chicken Pita (page 154)
or
Lean Cuisine Salmon with Basil

Dinner
Orecchiette with White Beans & Pesto (page 177)
or
Così Hummus & Veggie Sandwich

Snack #1
Pea & Walnut Hummus
(page 198)

Snack #2
Chocolate-Dipped Banana Bites
(page 212): Melt 2 tablespoons semisweet chocolate chips. Dip 1 small banana (peeled and cut into 1" chunks) in the chocolate.

FRIDAY (DAY 12)

Breakfast
Oatmeal with Prune & Banana Compote (page 128): Microwave ½ cup rolled oats with 1 cup low-fat milk for 3 to 5 minutes (according to package instructions). Top with 3 dried chopped plums, 1 diced banana, and 1 tablespoon chopped candied ginger.
or
Jamba Juice Fresh Banana Oatmeal

Lunch
Curried Egg Salad Sandwich
(page 142) plus 1 orange
or
Amy's Black Bean Vegetable Enchilada

Dinner
Bistro-Style Sirloin with New Potatoes (page 168)
or
P.F. Chang's Buddha's Feast steamed with a side of brown rice

Snack #1
Creamy Sweet Potato Dip
(page 204)

Snack #2
Quick Mango-Coconut Sorbet
(page 216)

SATURDAY (DAY 13)

Breakfast
Coconut French Toast with
Raspberry Syrup (page 126)
or
Orange Julius Bananarilla (20 ounces, medium)

Lunch
Chicken Pita Sandwich (page 102):
Toss 1 cup baby spinach, ½ cup sliced red bell pepper, and 4 ounces cooked boneless, skinless chicken strips with 2 tablespoons low fat Italian vinaigrette. Stuff into 1 (6") whole-grain pita (halved).
or
6" Subway Turkey Breast Sandwich on 9-grain wheat bread

Dinner
Bacon, Pear & Gorgonzola Pizza (page 194)
or
Lean Pockets Whole-Grain Grilled Chicken, Mushroom, and Spinach and a side salad

Snack #1
White Bean Salsa and Chips (page 199)

Snack #2
Raspberries with Chocolate Yogurt Mousse (page 224)

SUNDAY (DAY 14)

Breakfast
Broccoli & Feta Omelet with Toast (page 122)
or
Fiber One Blueberry Muffin plus 1 banana

Lunch
Greek Lentil Soup with Toasted Pita (page 145)
or
6" Subway Veggie Delite Sandwich on 9-grain wheat bread

Dinner
Baked Two-Cheese Penne with Roasted Red Pepper Sauce (page 192)
or
Amy's Southwestern Burrito and a side salad

Snack #1
Antipasto Platter (page 209):
12 canned black olives (drained), ½ cup marinated artichoke hearts (drained), and ½ red bell pepper (sliced).

Snack #2
Dark Chocolate & Oat Clusters (page 213)

21-Day Checklist Continued

■ **Don't be a slave (to your stove):** When life gets busy, opt for one of the Frozen Lunch and Dinner options (page 268) or a restaurant meal.

■ **Try exercising—even if you didn't before!** Carb-rich foods (such as those in our recipes in Chapter 7) slow digestion, which keeps glucose—the body's main energy source—pumping into your cells steadily. End result: Your energy never lags. No more sluggish afternoons. and lots more stamina for exercise.

MONDAY (DAY 15)

Breakfast
Polenta Fritters with Asparagus & Eggs (page 130)
or
6" Subway Egg & Cheese Sandwich on 9-grain wheat bread with egg white

Lunch
Pecan-Crusted Goat Cheese Salad with Pomegranate Vinaigrette (page 157)
or
Fazoli's Grilled Chicken Artichoke Salad

Dinner
Roasted Vegetables & Italian Sausage with Polenta (page 189)
or
Lean Cuisine Sun-Dried Tomato Pesto Chicken

Snack #1
Coconut-Date Truffles (page 196)

Snack #2:
Maple Brown Rice Pudding (page 219)

TUESDAY (DAY 16)

Breakfast
Toast with Walnut & Pear
Breakfast Spread (page 129): Blend
4 ounces low-fat cottage cheese until
smooth. Stir in 1 tablespoon chopped
walnuts and 1 diced pear. Serve on
2 slices toasted sourdough bread.
or
Jamba Juice Blueberry and Blackberry
Oatmeal

Lunch
Pesto Turkey Club (page 158):
Spread 2 teaspoons prepared pesto
onto 2 slices pumpernickel bread. Add
1 ounce sliced turkey, 1 slice cooked
turkey bacon, 2 romaine lettuce leaves,
and 4 slices tomato. Serve with 1 apple.
or
Così Hummus & Veggie Sandwich

Dinner
Seared Chicken Breasts with
French Potato Salad (page 185)
or
Amy's Mexican Tofu Scramble

Snack #1
Garlic & Herb Yogurt Dip
(page 201)

Snack #2
Merlot Strawberries with
Whipped Cream (page 220)

WEDNESDAY (DAY 17)

Breakfast
Apple & Almond Muesli (page 117):
Combine ½ cup rolled oats and
½ cup 1% low-fat milk in a small
bowl. Let stand 5 to 10 minutes. Stir
in 1 chopped apple, 2 tablespoons
sliced almonds, and 2 teaspoons
honey.
or
Aunt Jemima Great Starts Scrambled
Eggs & Bacon with Hash Brown
Potatoes

Lunch
Roast Beef Sandwich with
Horseradish Aïoli (page 161) plus
1 cup sliced cucumbers drizzled with
1 tablespoon low-fat Italian dressing.
or
Così Hummus & Veggie Sandwich

Dinner
Thai Peanut Noodles (page 190)
or
Healthy Choice Oven-Roasted Chicken

Snack #1
Sunflower Lentil Spread (page 203)

Snack #2
Sweet Potato Pudding (page 222)

THURSDAY (DAY 18)

Breakfast
Cornflakes, Low-Fat Milk & Berries (page 127): Combine 2 cups cornflakes and 1 cup 1% low-fat milk in a small bowl. Top with 1 cup fresh or thawed frozen berries.
or
Amy's Breakfast Burrito and 1 apple

Lunch
Red Grape & Tuna Salad Pita (page 159)
or
Panera Sierra Turkey Sandwich on Artisan Rye
or
Jamba Juice Chimichurri Chicken Wrap without sauce

Dinner
Grilled Burger & Three-Bean Salad (page 108)
or
Healthy Choice Café Steamers Chicken Pesto Classico

Snack #1
Creamy Sweet Potato Dip (page 204)

Snack #2
1 glass of red wine (5 ounces)

FRIDAY (DAY 19)

Breakfast
Oatmeal with Prune & Banana Compote (page 128): Combine 1 cup 1% low-fat milk and ½ cup rolled oats in a small microwave-safe bowl. Microwave on HIGH for 3 to 5 minutes (according to package directions). Top with 3 chopped dried plums, 1 diced banana, and 1 tablespoon chopped candied ginger.
or
Jamba Juice Fresh Banana Oatmeal

Lunch
Moroccan Chicken Pita (page 154)
or
P.F. Chang's Buddha's Feast, steamed, with a side of brown rice

Dinner
Shrimp Stir-Fry with Ginger (page 111)
or
Marie Callender's Honey-Roasted Turkey

Snack #1
Warm Pear with Cinnamon Ricotta (page 207)

Snack #2
3 Hershey's Special Dark miniatures

SATURDAY (DAY 20)

Breakfast
Sharp Cheddar & Egg on Rye
(page 134)
or
6" Subway Ham, Egg, & Cheese
on 9-grain bread with egg white

Lunch
**Indian Chicken Salad with
Peanuts** (page 149)
or
Healthy Choice Oven-Roasted Chicken

Dinner
Bacon, Pear & Gorgonzola Pizza
(page 194)
or
Chili's "Guiltless Grill" Grilled Chicken
Sandwich
or
Wendy's Southwest Taco Salad

Snack #1
White Bean Salsa and Chips
(page 199)

Snack #2
Tall (12-ounce) latte with
2% low-fat milk

SUNDAY (DAY 21)

Breakfast
**Blueberry Oat Pancakes with
Maple Yogurt** (page 120)
or
Amy's Breakfast Scramble Wrap

Lunch
Curried Egg Salad Sandwich
(page 142) plus 1 orange
or
Kashi Lemongrass Coconut Chicken

Dinner
**Skillet Salmon & Parmesan
Potatoes** (page 112)
or
Fazoli's Grilled Chicken Artichoke
Salad

Snack #1
Pistachio & Dried Cherry Crostini
(page 209): Combine 2 tablespoons
low-fat cottage cheese, 2 teaspoons
chopped pistachios, 2 teaspoons
chopped dried cherries, and 1 teaspoon honey. Serve on top of 2 rye
crispbread crackers.

Snack #2
Chocolate-Dipped Banana Bites
(page 212): Melt 2 tablespoons
semisweet chocolate chips. Dip 1
small banana (peeled and cut into
1-inch chunks) in melted chocolate.

"I Lost Weight on CarbLovers"

BEFORE

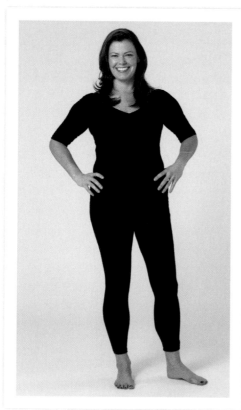

CHRISTY ELLINGER

Age: 38

Height: 5'8"

Weight before: 159

Weight after: 150

Pounds lost: 9

Biggest success: Seeing results outside of the scale. I've lost 10.5 inches, and my body is more toned.

Biggest challenge: Restaurant portions. *CarbLovers* taught me that meals in restaurants are too big. Now, if I order a steak, I'll eat half and take the rest home for later.

Favorite recipe: The Sirloin Salad with Blue Cheese Dressing & Sweet Potato Fries (page 181)—I love how indulgent that dinner is—beef, cheese, and fries just don't seem like diet food!

AFTER

I grew up eating food that wasn't healthy, and from time to time in my teen years I was an emotional eater: I didn't pay attention to what I was eating or drinking, and my weight would yo-yo.

As I got older it started to catch up with me. I was able to lose 20 pounds in college, but I hit a plateau, and ever since, I've found myself fighting to keep the same few from sneaking back on.

I tried a high-protein, low-carb diet for a week and felt disgusting from all the meat. I tried a shake-based diet, and I lost a lot of weight very quickly. Though I was happy with the results, I thought, 'Do I want to have shakes every day for the rest of my life?' No. I wanted a diet I could live with: Something that would keep those last persistent pounds off for good, and something sustainable.

I loved that *CarbLovers* wasn't very different from how I already ate. It simply taught me to look at the food on my plate before I eat, and make sure I've got the proportions right.

CarbLovers is great because it's not regimented. If I don't like a food, I don't have to eat it. And if there's something I want, nothing's off limits. If I want dessert, I have dessert! That kind of freedom made it easy for me. On top of that, I got the results I wanted. In just 12 weeks I lost 9 pounds. I feel like this plan is not just about short-term results—this is something I can incorporate into my everyday lifestyle.

Chapter 7

The *CarbLovers* Recipe Collection

WELCOME TO A NEW WORLD of delicious, real food. Meals you can look forward to each and every day for the rest of your life. Say goodbye forever to portions so small that your dinner was over and done with in just three bites, goodbye to snacks like rice cakes or even a handful of almonds (that never quite did it for me, either).

In the following pages, you'll find over 75 breakfast, lunch, dinner, snack, and dessert recipes. These sophisticated dishes are big on flavor, satisfaction, and metabolism-boosting oomph, but they are small on prep time and cost.

7-DAY *CARBLOVERS* KICKSTART RECIPES

BREAKFAST
Banana & Almond Butter Toast,
    page 95
Banana-Nut Oatmeal, page 96
Banana Shake, page 99

LUNCH
Big Chopped Salad, page 100
Chicken Pita Sandwich, page 102
Express Lunch Plate, page 103

DINNER
Black Bean Tacos, page 104
Chicken Pasta Primavera, page 107

Grilled Burger & Three-Bean Salad,
    page 108
Shrimp Stir-Fry with Ginger, page 111
Skillet Salmon & Parmesan Potatoes,
    page 112

SNACKS
Potato Chips, page 114
Black Beans & Chips, page 114
Trail Mix, page 114
Greek Yogurt Parfait, page 114
Almond Butter Crackers, page 114
White Bean & Herb Hummus with
    Crudités, page 115

HALLMARKS OF *CARBLOVERS* RECIPES

■ **They're loaded with Resistant Starch.** Main-course recipes include an average 3 grams of Resistant Starch (RS) each, and snacks average about 1 gram, making it easy for you to mix and match meals to hit your daily 10-gram target. (Look for RS in the nutritional analysis and in a yellow burst on the page.)

■ **Most of our recipes can be prepared in 20 minutes or less.** In fact, some take no time to make at all.

■ **They don't require special ingredients.** Nearly every item can be found at a grocery store near you—no matter where you live.

■ **They are affordable.** The ingredients used fit the budgets of even the most cost-conscious shopper.

Kickstart Breakfast Recipes

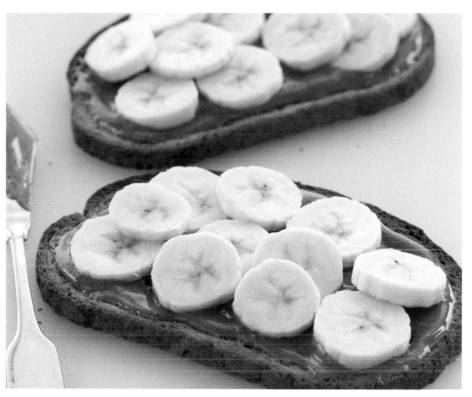

Banana & Almond Butter Toast

This breakfast option couldn't be simpler, but it packs a nutritional wallop. The rye bread and banana will get you halfway to your daily Resistant Starch goal, and the almond butter adds metabolism-boosting MUFAs.

Resistant Starch: 5.6g

PREP: 5 minutes
TOTAL TIME: 5 minutes
MAKES: 1 serving

> 1 **tablespoon almond butter**
> 1 **slice rye bread, toasted**
> 1 **banana, sliced**

1. Spread almond butter on toast.

2. Top with banana slices.

Serving size: 1½ cups | Calories 280; Fat 11g (sat 1g, mono 7g, poly 2.5g); Cholesterol 0mg; Protein 6g; Carbohydrate 44g; Sugars 16g; Fiber 5g; RS 5.6g; Sodium 260mg

Banana-Nut Oatmeal

By combining Resistant Starch powerhouses—banana and oatmeal—this morning meal alone gets you halfway to your Resistant Starch goal of 10 daily grams. The walnuts add some omega-3s, too, for extra fat-burning.

PREP: 5 minutes
COOK: 5 minutes
TOTAL TIME: 10 minutes
MAKES: 1 serving

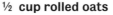

Resistant Starch:
5.2g

½ **cup rolled oats**
1 **cup water**
1 **banana, sliced**
1 **tablespoon chopped walnuts**
1 **teaspoon cinnamon**

1. Combine oats and 1 cup water in a small microwave-safe bowl. Microwave at HIGH 3 minutes.

2. Top with banana slices, walnuts, and cinnamon.

Serving size: 1½ cups | Calories 310; Fat 8g (sat 1g, mono 1.5g, poly 4.5g); Cholesterol 0mg; Protein 8g; Carbohydrate 57g; Sugars 16g; Fiber 9g; RS 5.2g; Sodium 0mg

★ CarbStar! ★
OATMEAL
4.6 grams of Resistant Starch per ½ cup raw or toasted oats

Oatmeal for breakfast might help you eat less all day. In a series of experiments, researchers in Italy replaced the flour in bread and pasta with oats. They found that even when these foods had identical calorie counts, oat eaters consumed fewer calories over the course of the day.

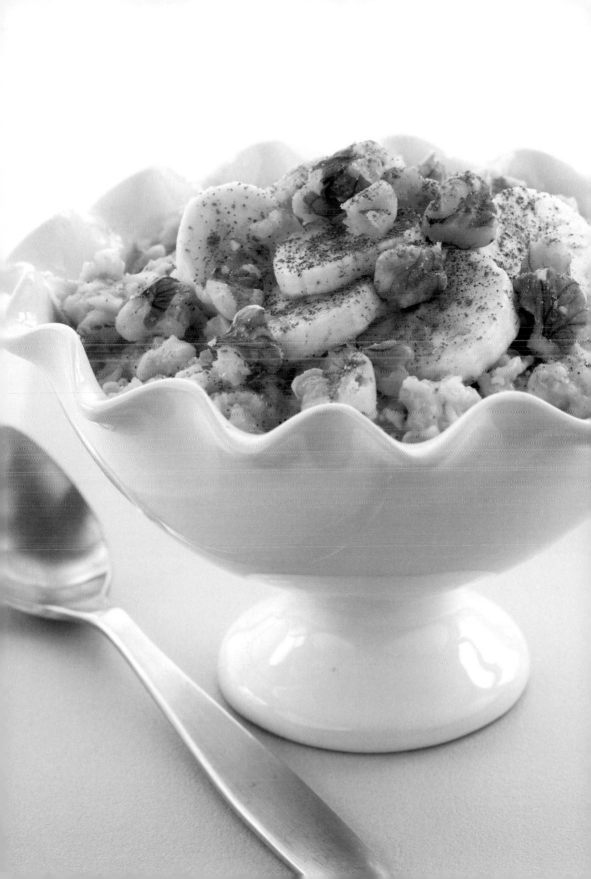

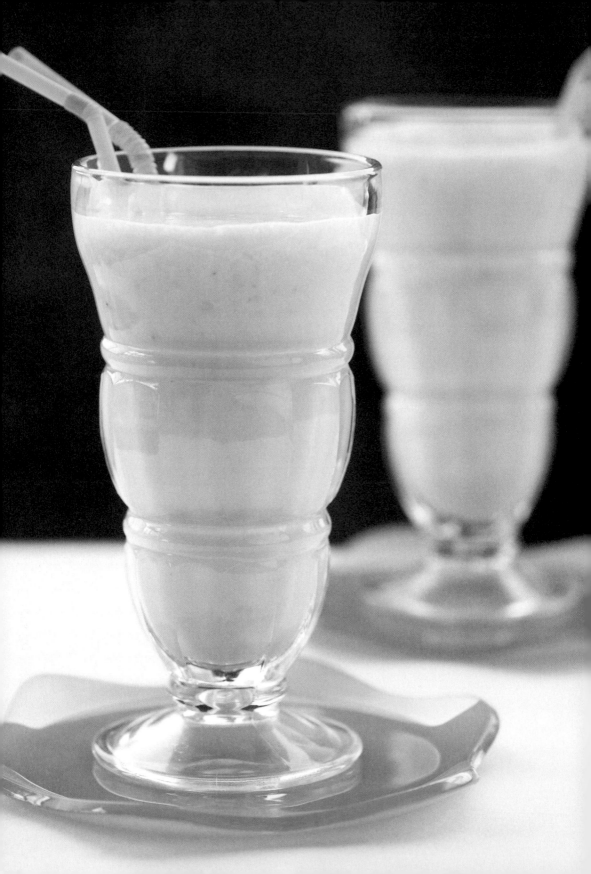

Banana Shake

Need a Resistant Starch shortcut? Eat a banana. It's the secret reason this shake is such a slimming way to start your morning. If you're not a breakfast eater, shakes are also an easy way to get the Resistant Starch you need without feeling stuffed.

Resistant Starch: 4.7g

PREP: 5 minutes
TOTAL TIME: 5 minutes
MAKES: 1 serving

- 1 banana
- 1½ cups 1% low-fat milk
- 2 teaspoons honey
- ½ cup ice

1. Place all ingredients in a blender; process until smooth.

Serving size: 1½ cups | Calories 300; Fat 4g (sat 2.5g, mono 1g, poly 0g); Cholesterol 20mg; Protein 14g; Carbohydrate 57g; Sugars 44g; Fiber 3g; RS 4.7g; Sodium 170mg

Variations:
Banana Shake Plus: Add 2 teaspoons ground flaxseed.
Banana-Cocoa Shake: Add 1 tablespoon unsweetened cocoa.
Banana-Berry Shake: Add ¼ cup berries (any variety).

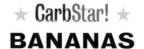

★ CarbStar! ★
BANANAS

4.7 to 12.5 grams of Resistant Starch per serving, depending on ripeness

Bananas are your richest source of Resistant Starch, with ripe ones offering 4.7 grams of the fat flusher and less ripe (slightly green) bananas containing a whopping 12.5 grams. They are also rich in appetite-suppressing fiber (with 3 grams per 1 medium banana) and contain the amino acid tryptophan, which is converted into the calming brain chemical serotonin to relax and improve your mood.

Kickstart Lunch Recipes

Big Chopped Salad

You can build this at any salad bar or make it yourself from ingredients you have at home. This salad provides nearly half of your daily fiber, thanks in part to the garbanzo beans.

Resistant Starch:
2.1g

PREP: 5 minutes
TOTAL TIME: 5 minutes
MAKES: 1 serving

    3   cups mixed salad greens
    ½   cup canned no-salt-added garbanzo
        beans, rinsed and drained
    ½   cup shredded carrots
    ½   cup shredded red cabbage
    1   tablespoon grated Parmesan cheese
    2   tablespoons chopped walnuts
    2   tablespoons dried cranberries
    2   tablespoons low-fat balsamic
        vinaigrette

1. Combine first 7 ingredients (through cranberries) in a large bowl.

2. Toss with vinaigrette and serve.

Serving size: 4½ cups | Calories 390; Fat 14g (sat 2g, mono 2g, poly 8g); Cholesterol 5mg; Protein 15g; Carbohydrate 60g; Sugars 23g; Fiber 13g; RS 2.1g; Sodium 630mg

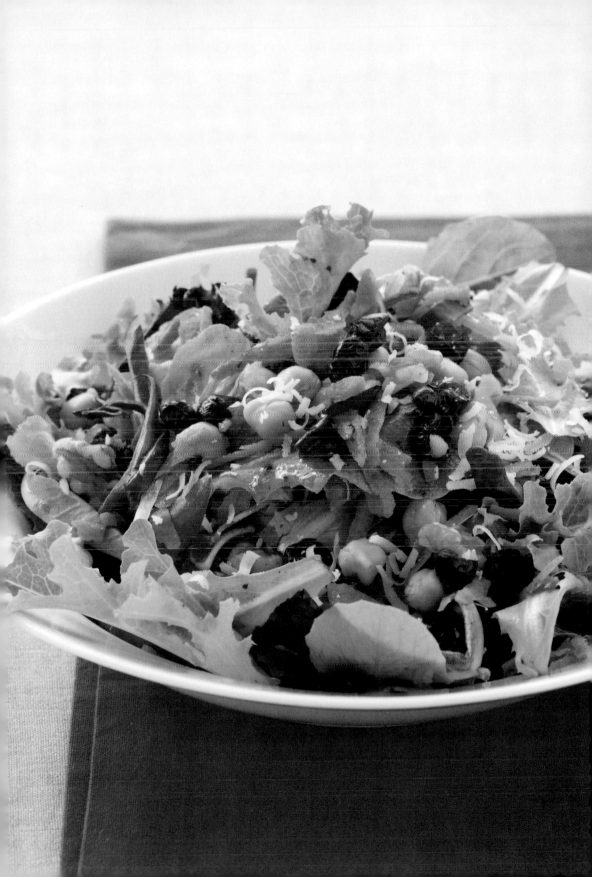

Chicken Pita Sandwich

This easy sandwich will fill you up with lean protein, along with a hearty 5 grams of fiber from the whole-grain pita and veggies inside. Use precooked chicken strips or rotisserie chicken to save time.

PREP: 5 minutes
TOTAL TIME: 5 minutes
MAKES: 1 serving

- 1 **cup baby spinach**
- ½ **cup (4 ounces) cooked skinless, boneless chicken breast, sliced into ½-inch strips**
- ½ **cup sliced red bell pepper**
- 2 **tablespoons low-fat Italian vinaigrette**
- 1 **(6-inch) whole-grain pita, cut in half**

1. Combine spinach, chicken, bell pepper, and vinaigrette in a bowl; toss gently.

2. Serve in pita halves.

Serving size: 2 stuffed pita halves | Calories 400; Fat 10g (sat 1.5g, mono 1.5g, poly 2g); Cholesterol 95mg; Protein 43g; Carbohydrate 36g; Sugars 5g; Fiber 6g; RS 1g; Sodium 670mg

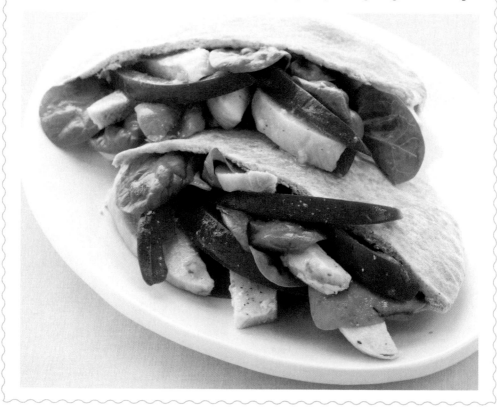

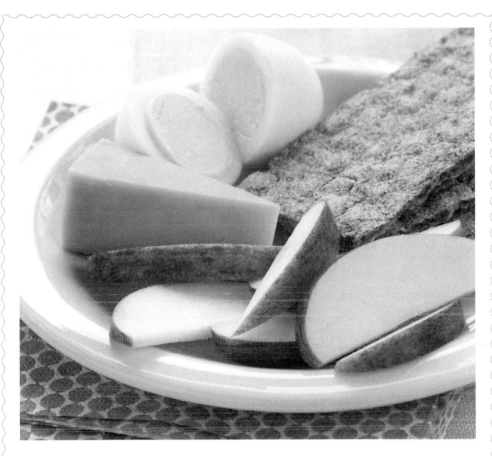

Express Lunch Plate

Grab the ingredients for this fast, filling lunch from the corner deli. This combo is rich in fiber, protein, and other metabolism boosters. If you prefer a different type of cheese, swap it.

PREP: 5 minutes
TOTAL TIME: 5 minutes
MAKES: 1 serving

Resistant Starch:

1g

- 1 **large hard-cooked egg**
- 1 **(1-ounce) Cheddar cheese wedge**
- 1 **apple, cored and sliced**
- 3 **rye crispbread crackers**

1. Arrange all ingredients on a plate and enjoy.

Serving size: 1 plate | Calories 400; Fat 15g (sat 8g, mono 5g, poly 1g); Cholesterol 240mg; Protein 16g; Carbohydrate 51g; Sugars 20g; Fiber 9g; RS 1g; Sodium 320mg

Kickstart Dinner Recipes

Black Bean Tacos

The black beans in this dish should be every dieter's best friend. They provide plenty of Resistant Starch, along with appetite suppressing fiber and protein. The cheese offers CLA for an extra metabolism kick. To save time, use prewashed lettuce and preshredded carrots.

Resistant Starch: 4.7g

PREP: 5 minutes
COOK: 5 minutes
TOTAL TIME: 10 minutes
MAKES: 2 servings

- 1 (15-ounce) can no-salt–added black beans, rinsed and drained
- 6 (6-inch) corn tortillas
- 6 tablespoons shredded Cheddar cheese
- 2 cups shredded Romaine lettuce
- 1 cup grated carrots
- ¼ cup salsa

1. Microwave beans at HIGH 2 minutes or until heated through.

2. Heat a nonstick skillet over medium heat. Add tortillas, one at a time; cook 1 minute on each side.

3. Divide beans evenly among tortillas. Top with even amounts of cheese, lettuce, carrot, and salsa.

Serving size: 3 tacos | Calories 420; Fat 8g (sat 5g, mono 0.5g, poly 1g); Cholesterol 25mg; Protein 18g; Carbohydrate 69g; Sugars 5g; Fiber 17g; RS 4.7g; Sodium 420mg

★ CarbStar! ★
BEANS
1.5 to 3.8 grams of Resistant Starch per serving

Nearly half of the starch in beans comes from Resistant Starch, making them a powerful weight-loss ally. They are also an incredibly rich source of fiber, providing 15 grams per cup. It's no wonder that a Canadian study of 1,475 men and women found that those who consumed beans regularly tended to weigh less and have a smaller waist circumference than those who did not eat them. They were also 23 percent less likely to become overweight over time.

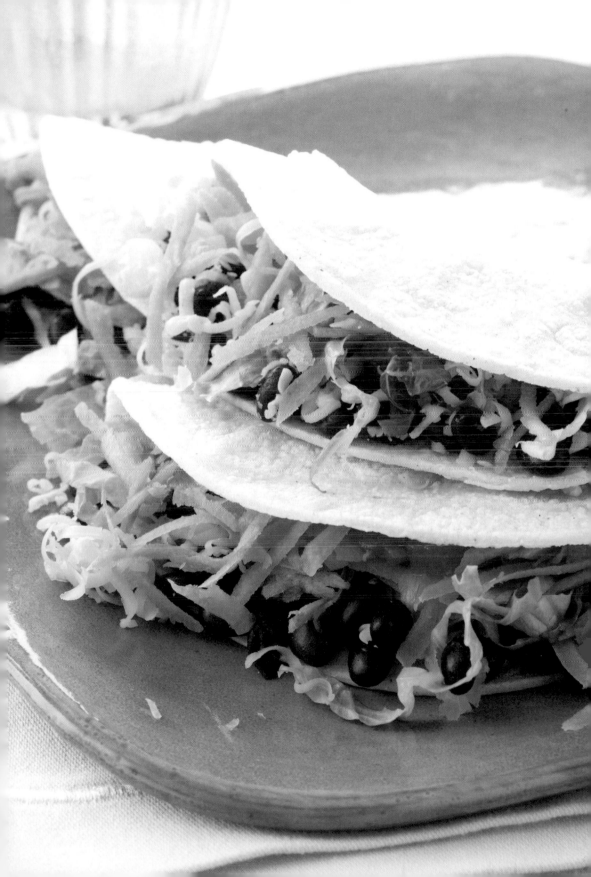

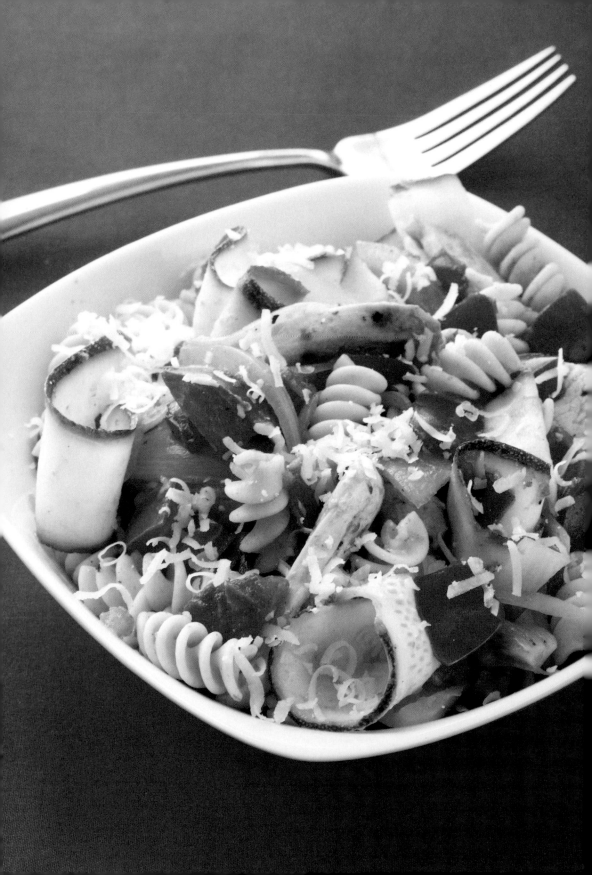

Chicken Pasta Primavera

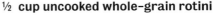

To save time, batch-cook the pasta and use precooked or rotisserie chicken for this easy, fiber-packed dish. Use a vegetable peeler to make the zucchini ribbons.

PREP: 5 minutes
COOK: 15 minutes
TOTAL TIME: 20 minutes
MAKES: 2 servings

Resistant Starch: 2 g

- ½ cup uncooked whole-grain rotini
- 2 teaspoons olive oil
- ½ cup (4 ounces) cooked skinless, boneless chicken breast, sliced into ½-inch strips
- 1 onion, vertically sliced
- 3 garlic cloves, minced
- 1 teaspoon dried oregano
- ⅛ teaspoon salt
- ⅛ teaspoon pepper
- 2 cups chopped tomato
- 1 zucchini, sliced lengthwise into ribbons
- 2 tablespoons grated Parmesan cheese

1. Cook pasta according to package directions, omitting salt and fat. Drain.

2. Heat oil in a nonstick skillet over medium heat. Add chicken; cook 5 minutes.

3. Add onion, garlic, oregano, salt, pepper, and tomato to pan; cook 8–10 minutes.

4. Combine chicken mixture, pasta, and zucchini ribbons; toss gently. Top with Parmesan cheese.

Serving size: 3½ cups | Calories 410; Fat 9g (sat 2g, mono 3.5g, poly 1g); Cholesterol 40mg; Protein 28g; Carbohydrate 61g; Sugars 13g; Fiber 12g; RS 2g; Sodium 480mg

Grilled Burger & Three-Bean Salad

With 29 grams of protein, this is a stick-to-your-ribs meal that—thanks to plenty of metabolism boosters—will fill you up but won't fill you out.

PREP: 5 minutes
COOK: 15 minutes
TOTAL TIME: 20 minutes
MAKES: 2 servings

Resistant Starch: **2.3**g

- 6 **ounces lean ground sirloin or bison**
- 1 **teaspoon olive oil**
- ½ **cup green beans, fresh or frozen, thawed**
- ½ **cup canned white beans, rinsed and drained**
- ½ **cup canned kidney beans, rinsed and drained**
- ½ **cup carrot, peeled and chopped**
- ½ **cup chopped green bell pepper**
- 2 **(1½-ounce) whole-grain hamburger buns**
- 2 **tablespoons low-fat Italian vinaigrette**
  Romaine lettuce leaves
- 4 **tomato slices**

1. Divide beef into 2 equal portions, shaping each into a ½-inch-thick patty.

2. Heat oil in a nonstick skillet over medium heat. Place patties in pan; cook 6 minutes each side or until a meat thermometer inserted into middle of burger reads 160°.

3. Combine green beans, white beans, kidney beans, carrot, bell pepper, and vinaigrette in a bowl; toss gently.

4. On the bottom of each bun, place a few lettuce leaves and 2 slices tomato; top with burger and other half of bun. Serve bean salad alongside burgers.

Serving size: 1 burger and 1 cup salad | Calories 400; Fat 11g (sat 2g, mono 4g, poly 2g); Cholesterol 45mg; Protein 29g; Carbohydrate 50g; Sugars 9g; Fiber 12g; RS 2.3g; Sodium 580mg

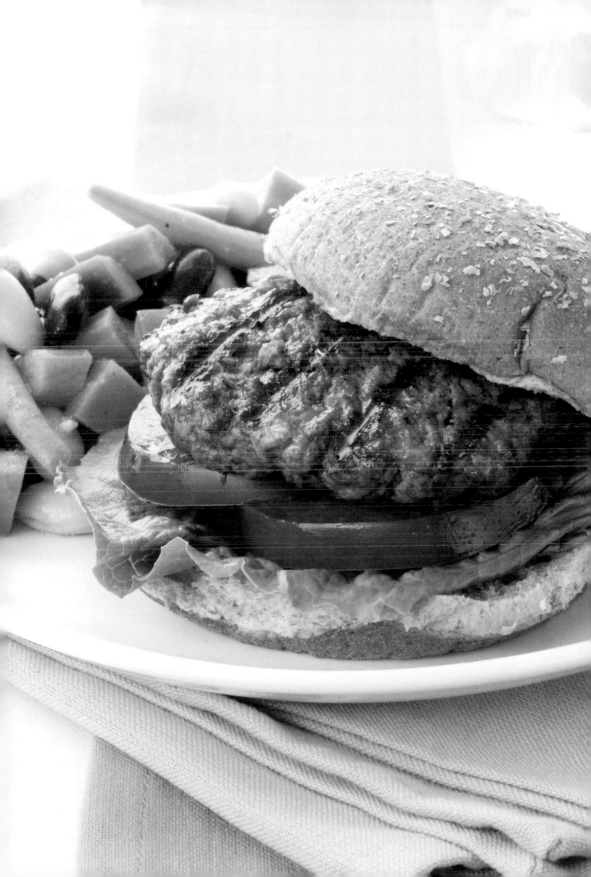

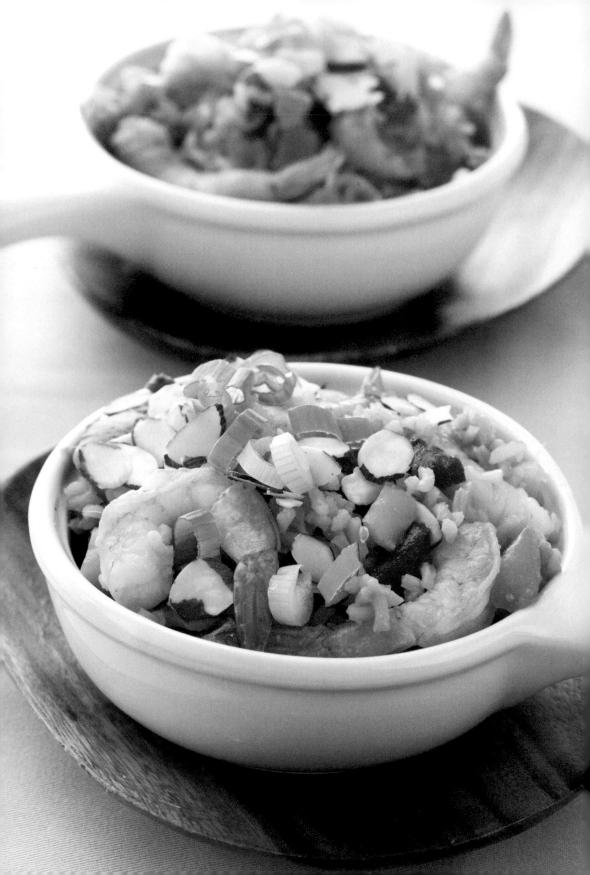

Shrimp Stir-Fry with Ginger

To save time, use a fast-cooking brown rice (such as Uncle Ben's Fast & Natural Whole Grain Brown Rice) to get this crowd-pleasing meal on the table even faster.

PREP: 5 minutes
COOK: 10 minutes
TOTAL TIME: 15 minutes
MAKES: 2 servings

Resistant Starch:
2.6g

- 2 teaspoons dark sesame oil
- 2 tablespoons less-sodium soy sauce
- 1 tablespoon honey
- 1 tablespoon grated peeled fresh ginger
- 2 garlic cloves, minced
- 4 cups frozen stir-fry vegetables, thawed
- 3 ounces (about 14 medium) frozen precooked shrimp, thawed
- 1½ cups cooked brown rice
- 2 tablespoons sliced almonds
- 1 scallion, chopped

1. Heat oil in a large nonstick skillet over medium heat. Add soy sauce, honey, ginger, and garlic; cook 1 minute.

2. Add vegetables, shrimp, and cooked rice; cook 8 minutes.

3. Remove from heat. Top with almonds and scallions.

Serving size: 3 cups | Calories 410; Fat 9g (sat 1.5g, mono 4g, poly 3.5g); Cholesterol 65mg; Protein 17g; Carbohydrate 61g; Sugars 14g; Fiber 6g; RS 2.6g; Sodium 710mg

Skillet Salmon & Parmesan Potatoes

Salmon, like tuna, is packed with metabolism-boosting omega-3 fatty acids. This dish also features CLA in the cheese, Resistant Starch from the potatoes, and fiber from the greens.

PREP: 8 minutes
COOK: 12 minutes
TOTAL TIME: 20 minutes
MAKES: 2 servings

1 (6-ounce) salmon fillet (about 1-inch thick)
  Cooking spray
2 medium potatoes
  Salt and pepper, to taste
4 tablespoons shredded Parmesan cheese
2 cups mixed salad greens
1 cup chopped tomatoes
2 tablespoons low-fat balsamic vinaigrette
1 lemon

1. Heat a nonstick skillet or grill pan over medium-high heat. Coat fish with cooking spray. Add fish to pan, and cook 6 minutes on each side or until fish flakes easily when tested with a fork.

2. While fish cooks, pierce potatoes with a fork; arrange in a circle on paper towels in a microwave oven. Microwave at HIGH 8–10 minutes, turning potatoes after 5 minutes. Let stand 5 minutes.

3. Cut the cooked potatoes in half, and sprinkle with the salt, pepper, and Parmesan cheese.

4. Combine greens, tomatoes, and vinaigrette in a bowl; toss gently.

5. Cut lemon in half, and squeeze lemon juice over fish. Serve salmon with potatoes and salad.

Serving size: 3 ounces salmon, 2 potato halves, and 1½ cups salad | Calories 410; Fat 12g (sat 3g, mono 2g, poly 2g); Cholesterol 50mg; Protein 30g; Carbohydrate 49g; Sugars 7g; Fiber 7g; RS 2.1g; Sodium 660mg

★ CarbStar! ★

POTATOES

1 to 3.7 grams of Resistant Starch

In addition to fiber and Resistant Starch, potatoes are a natural source of a proteinase inhibitor, a natural chemical that boosts satiety hormones and curbs appetite. Potatoes are also incredibly filling and—at 300 calories for a large, baked spud—great for weight loss.

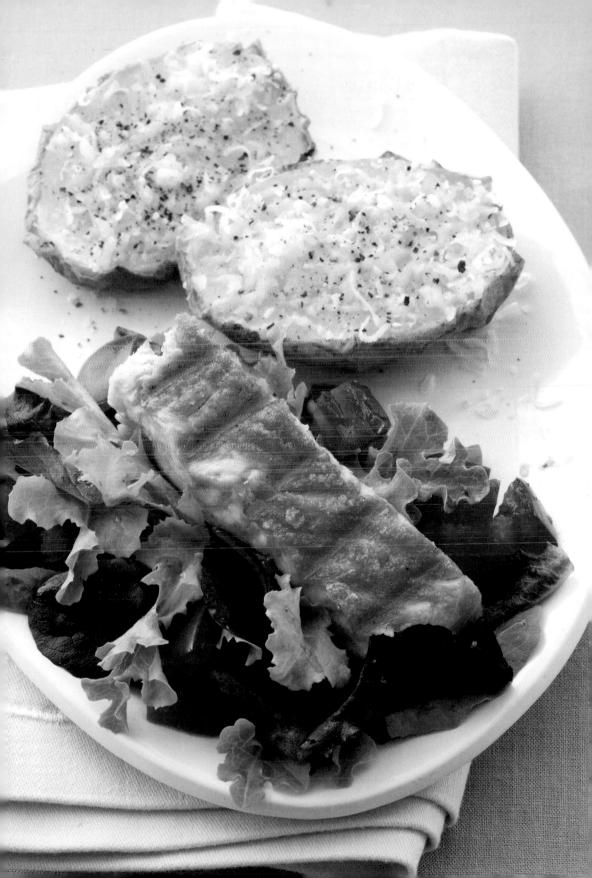

Kickstart Snacks

**During Phase 1, you can choose one snack a day.
Try one of these:**

- White Bean & Herb Hummus with Crudités (shown at right)

- Potato chips: Crunch on 24 chips (about 1 ounce).

- Black Beans & Chips: Enjoy 2 tablespoons canned black beans, rinsed and drained, with 8 corn tortilla chips.

- Trail Mix: Combine ½ cup cornflakes, 2 tablespoons sliced almonds, and 2 tablespoons dried cherries.

- Greek Yogurt Parfait: Top ¾ cup (6 ounces) plain low-fat Greek yogurt with 2 teaspoons honey and 2 tablespoons old-fashioned rolled oats, uncooked or toasted.

- Almond Butter Crackers: Nosh on 2 teaspoons almond butter spread on 2 rye crispbread crackers.

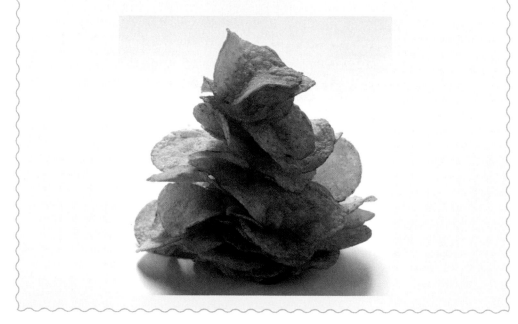

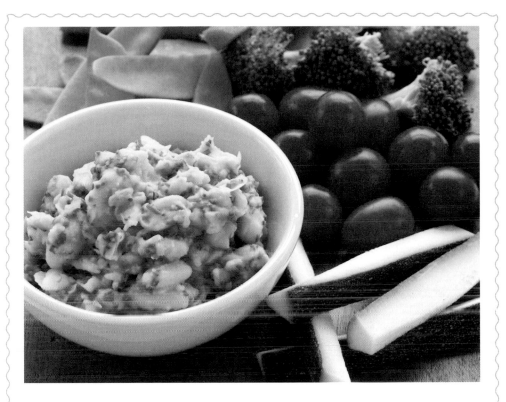

White Bean & Herb Hummus with Crudités

The MUFAs, fiber, and Resistant Starch in this snack will tide you over until your next meal.

PREP: 5 minutes
TOTAL TIME: 5 minutes
MAKES: 1 serving

Resistant Starch: 2 g

¼ **cup canned white beans, rinsed and drained**
1 **tablespoon chopped chives**
1 **tablespoon lemon juice**
2 **teaspoons olive oil**
½ **cup assorted raw vegetables, such as chopped broccoli florets, cherry tomatoes, zucchini spears, and sugar snap peas**

1. Combine beans, chives, lemon juice, and oil in a small bowl. Mash with a fork until mixture thickens but still has texture.

2. Serve with raw vegetables.

Serving size: ¼ cup hummus and ½ cup raw vegetables |
Calories 150; Fat 10g (sat 1.5g, mono 7g, poly 1g); Cholesterol 0mg; Protein 4g; Carbohydrate 14g; Sugars 3g; Fiber 3g; RS 2g; Sodium 35mg

21-DAY IMMERSION RECIPES

Immersion Breakfast Recipes

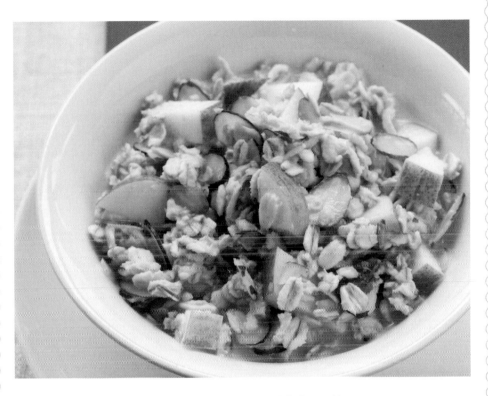

Apple & Almond Muesli

If mornings are hectic for you, make this dish the day before. Mix all of the ingredients, cover, and refrigerate overnight.

PREP: 5 minutes
STAND: 7 minutes
TOTAL TIME: 12 minutes
MAKES: 1 serving

½ **cup old-fashioned rolled oats**
½ **cup 1% low-fat milk**
1 **apple, cored and chopped**
2 **tablespoons sliced almonds**
2 **teaspoons honey**

1. Combine oats and milk in a small bowl; let stand 7 minutes.

2. Stir in apple, almonds, and honey.

Serving size: 2 cups | Calories 400; Fat 10g (sat 2g, mono 5g, poly 2.5g); Cholesterol 5mg; Protein 12g; Carbohydrate 72g; Sugars 38g; Fiber 10g; RS 4.6g; Sodium 55mg

Banana Yogurt Parfait with Maple Oat Topping

Uncooked oats offer four times as much Resistant Starch as cooked, which is why this recipe calls for you to only lightly toast them.

PREP: 5 minutes
COOK: 5 minutes
TOTAL TIME: 10 minutes
MAKES: 1 serving

Resistant Starch: **8.2** g

- 6 tablespoons old-fashioned rolled oats
- 1 tablespoon pure maple syrup
- ¾ cup plain low-fat Greek yogurt
- 1 banana, sliced

1. Heat a nonstick skillet over medium heat. In a small bowl, combine oats and maple syrup; add oat mixture to pan, and cook 2–3 minutes.

2. Place yogurt in a bowl and top with banana and toasted oats.

Serving size: 1½ cups | Calories 380; Fat 6g (sat 3g, mono 1g, poly 1g); Cholesterol 10mg; Protein 19g; Carbohydrate 67g; Sugars 34g; Fiber 6g; RS 8.2g; Sodium 60mg

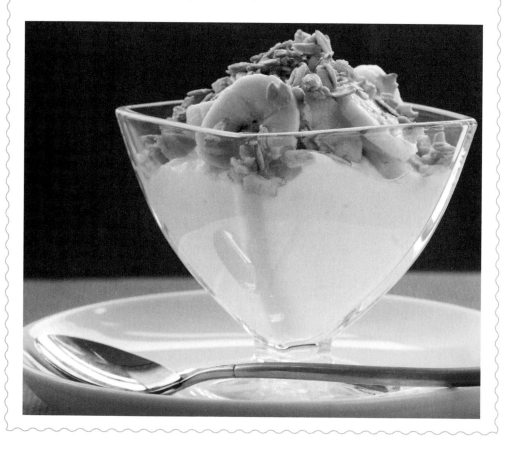

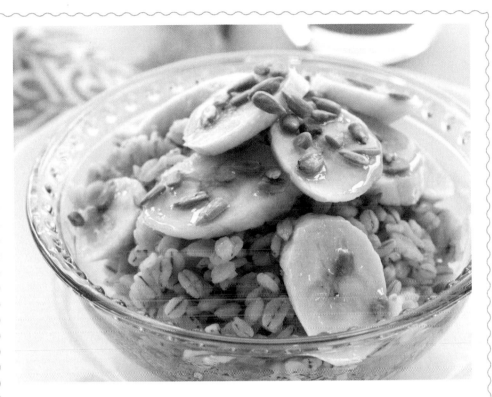

Breakfast Barley with Banana & Sunflower Seeds

With a whopping 7.6 grams of Resistant Starch plus some metabolism-boosting fiber and MUFAs, to boot, this is an ultrasatisfying morning meal.

PREP: 5 minutes
COOK: 10 minutes
TOTAL TIME: 15 minutes
MAKES: 1 serving

Resistant Starch: 7.6 g

⅔ **cup water**
⅓ **cup uncooked quick-cooking pearl barley**
1 **banana, sliced**
1 **teaspoon honey**
1 **tablespoon unsalted sunflower seeds**

1. Combine water and barley in a small microwave-safe bowl. Microwave at HIGH 6 minutes.

2. Stir and let stand 2 minutes.

3. Top with banana slices, honey, and sunflower seeds.

Serving size: 1 cup | Calories 410; Fat 6g (sat 0.5g, mono 2g, poly 2.5g); Cholesterol 0mg; Protein 10g; Carbohydrate 86g; Sugars 21g; Fiber 14g; RS 7.6g; Sodium 15mg

Blueberry Oat Pancakes with Maple Yogurt

Because this dish takes some time to prepare, save it for a weekend morning when you're not in a rush. If you can't find Greek yogurt, substitute plain low-fat yogurt instead. You can use either fresh or thawed frozen unsweetened berries.

PREP: 5 minutes
COOK: 10 minutes
TOTAL TIME: 15 minutes
MAKES: 2 servings

Resistant Starch:

4.6g

1 **cup old-fashioned rolled oats**
½ **cup low-fat cottage cheese**
2 **large eggs**
1 **teaspoon vanilla extract**
1 **cup blueberries**
  Cooking spray
¾ **cup plain low-fat Greek yogurt**
1 **tablespoon maple syrup**

1. Combine oats, cottage cheese, eggs, and vanilla in a blender or food processor; process until smooth. Gently stir in the blueberries.

2. Heat a large nonstick skillet over medium heat. Coat pan with cooking spray. Spoon about 2 tablespoons batter per pancake into pan. Cook 3 minutes or until tops are covered with bubbles and edges look cooked. Carefully turn pancakes over, and cook 3 more minutes or until golden.

3. Combine yogurt and maple syrup; serve alongside pancakes.

Serving size: 3 (3-inch) pancakes and about ½ cup yogurt mixture | Calories 410; Fat 12g (sat 3.5g, mono 3g, poly 2g); Cholesterol 220mg; Protein 26g; Carbohydrate 50g; Sugars 20g; Fiber 6g; RS 4.6g; Sodium 330mg

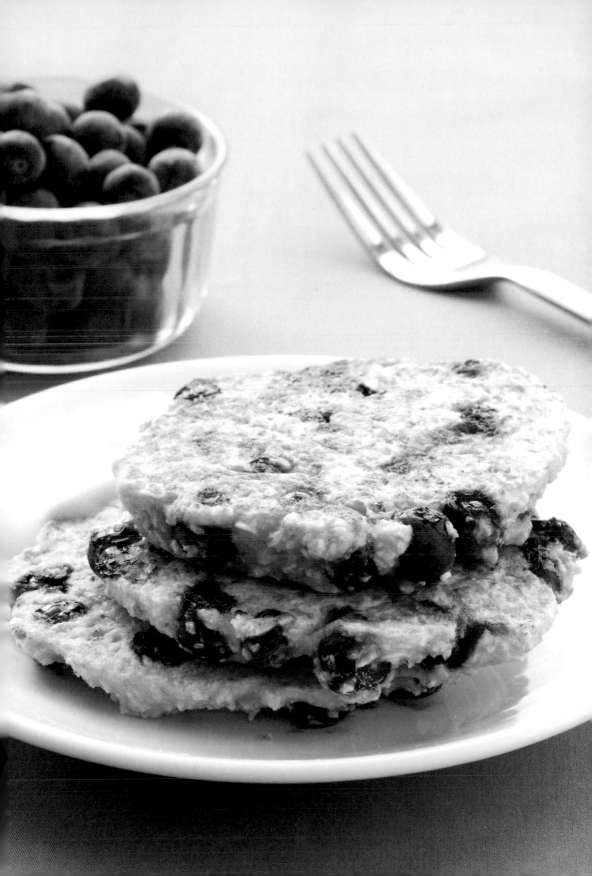

Broccoli & Feta Omelet with Toast

Who needs breakfast at a diner when you can whip up a dish like this in no time flat? Use either fresh or frozen broccoli—both work just fine. The Feta cheese adds some CLA plus a punch of flavor, too.

PREP: 5 minutes
COOK: 10 minutes
TOTAL TIME: 15 minutes
MAKES: 1 serving

Resistant Starch:
1.8 g

    Cooking spray
1 **cup chopped broccoli**
2 **large eggs, whisked**
2 **tablespoons Feta cheese, crumbled**
¼ **teaspoon dried dill**
2 **slices rye bread, toasted**

1. Heat a nonstick skillet over medium heat. Coat pan with cooking spray. Add broccoli, and cook 3 minutes.

2. Combine eggs, Feta, and dill in a small bowl. Add egg mixture to pan. Cook 3–4 minutes; fold in half with a spatula and cook 2 more minutes or until cooked through. Serve with toast.

Serving size: 1 omelet and 2 pieces toast | Calories 390; Fat 19g (sat 6g, mono 5g, poly 2g); Cholesterol 440mg; Protein 23g; Carbohydrate 35g; Sugars 5g; Fiber 6g; RS 1.8g; Sodium 550mg

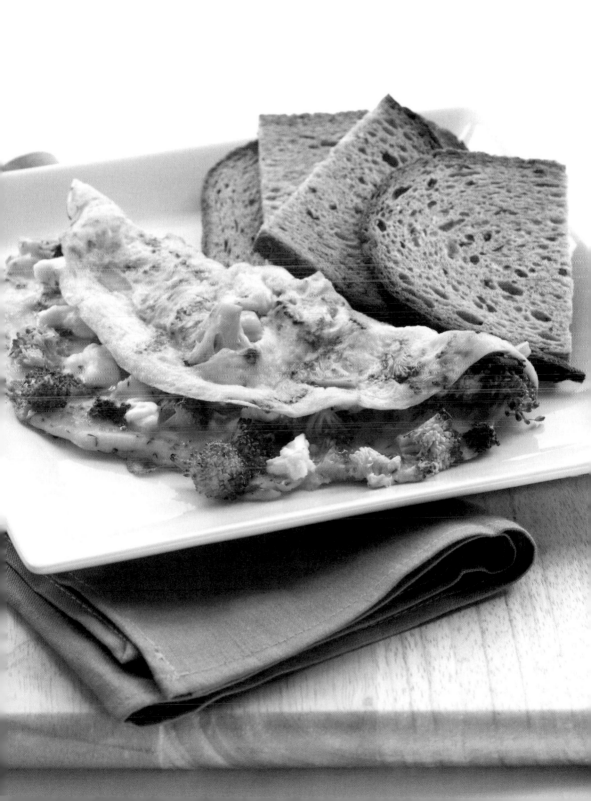

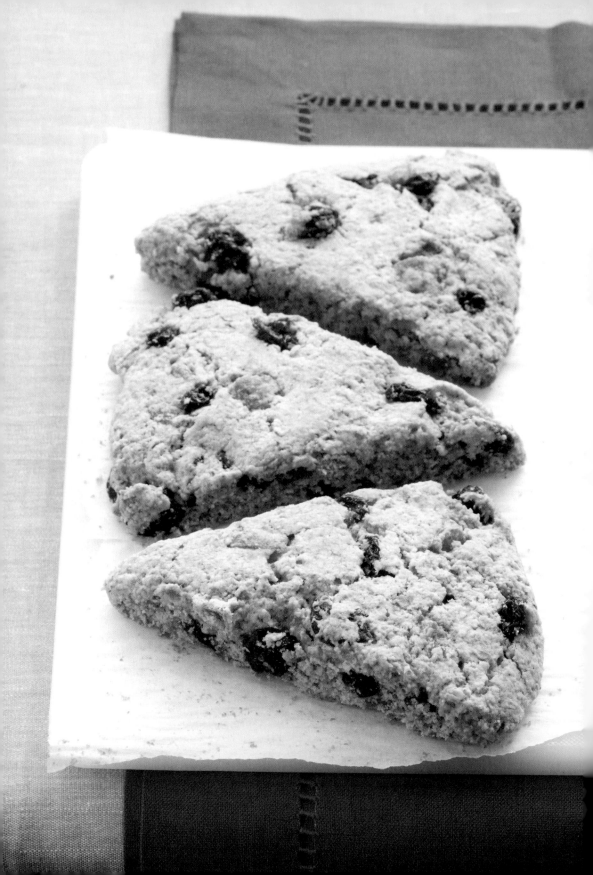

Cherry-Ginger Scones

Bet you never thought you'd be eating scones while you were on a diet! These scones, however, are so diet friendly that they aren't even a dessert—you can have them for breakfast. High in fiber, protein, and Resistant Starch, they will keep you satisfied in every way.

PREP: 20 minutes
BAKE: 25 minutes
TOTAL TIME: 45 minutes
MAKES: 8 servings

Resistant Starch:
1.2 g

- 1½ cups whole-wheat pastry flour
- 1 cup old-fashioned rolled oats
- ¼ cup packed brown sugar
- 2 teaspoons baking powder
- ½ teaspoon baking soda
- ¼ teaspoon salt
- ½ cup unsalted butter
- 1 cup dried cherries
- ½ cup crystallized ginger, coarsely chopped
- ¼ cup low-fat buttermilk
- 2 large egg whites, whisked
  All-purpose flour (as needed)

1. Preheat oven to 350°. Line a baking sheet with parchment paper, and set aside.

2. Combine flour, oats, brown sugar, baking powder, baking soda, and salt in a food processor. Process 10 seconds or until oats are finely chopped. Add butter; process until mixture resembles coarse meal.

3. Transfer flour mixture to a large mixing bowl; stir in cherries and crystallized ginger.

4. Combine buttermilk and egg whites in a small bowl; stir with a whisk. Add buttermilk mixture to flour mixture; stir just until a sticky dough forms.

5. Transfer dough to parchment paper lined baking sheet, and pat into a 9-inch circle (about 1-inch thick). Sprinkle with all-purpose flour, if necessary, to keep the dough from sticking to hands. Divide the dough into 8 equal wedges. Separate wedges slightly, and bake at 350° for 25 minutes or until golden brown and a wooden pick inserted in center comes out clean.

Serving size: 1 scone | Calories 348; Fat 13g (sat 7.5g, mono 3g, poly 1g); Cholesterol 31mg; Protein 6g; Carbohydrate 53g; Sugars 20g; Fiber 5g; RS 1.2g; Sodium 271mg

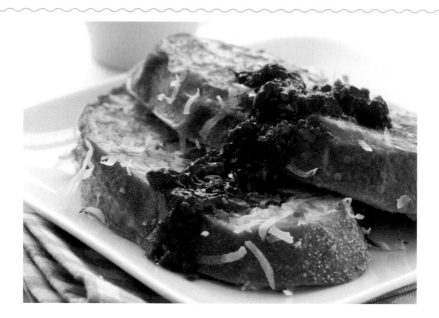

Coconut French Toast with Raspberry Syrup

Save this delicious dish for a weekend morning when you are not in a rush. You can use fresh or thawed frozen unsweetened raspberries.

PREP: 5 minutes
COOK: 10 minutes
TOTAL TIME: 15 minutes
MAKES: 2 servings

Resistant Starch:
1.2 g

   2 **large eggs**
  ½ **cup 1% low-fat milk**
   1 **teaspoon vanilla extract**
   4 **(½-inch-thick) slices sourdough bread**
   2 **tablespoons shredded coconut**
     Cooking spray
   1 **cup raspberries**
   2 **tablespoons pure maple syrup**

1. In a large bowl, whisk together eggs, milk, and vanilla.

2. Lightly dip bread slices in egg mixture; pat shredded coconut onto both sides of bread.

3. Heat a large nonstick skillet over medium heat. Coat pan with cooking spray. Add bread slices; cook 4 minutes on each side or until golden.

4. Combine raspberries and maple syrup in a small microwave-safe bowl. Microwave at HIGH 30 seconds. Serve over French toast.

Serving size: 2 pieces French toast and 4 tablespoons syrup |
Calories 410; Fat 12g (sat 5g, mono 2.5g, poly 1.5g); Cholesterol 215mg; Protein 16g; Carbohydrate 58g; Sugars 20g; Fiber 6g; RS 1.2g; Sodium 470mg

Cornflakes, Low-Fat Milk & Berries

It doesn't matter what types of berries you use for this recipe. All of them—strawberries, blueberries, raspberries, blackberries—are high in fiber, low in calories, and rich in antioxidants.

PREP: 5 minutes
TOTAL TIME: 5 minutes
MAKES: 1 serving

Resistant Starch: 1.8 g

2 cups cornflakes
1 cup 1% low-fat milk
1 cup berries, fresh or frozen, thawed

1. Place cornflakes in a small bowl. Top with milk and berries.

Serving size: 3 cups | Calories 370; Fat 3g (sat 1.5g, mono 1g, poly 0g); Cholesterol 10mg; Protein 13g; Carbohydrate 78g; Sugars 27g; Fiber 6g; RS 1.8g; Sodium 640mg

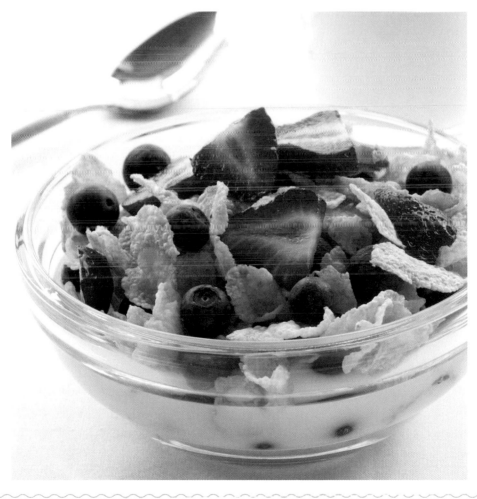

Oatmeal with Prune & Banana Compote

A rich source of vitamin C and polyphenols (a type of antioxidant thought to protect brain cells from damage), dried plums—which you may know as prunes—add rich flavor to this traditional morning dish.

PREP: 5 minutes
COOK: 5 minutes
TOTAL TIME: 10 minutes
MAKES: 1 serving

Resistant Starch:

5.2g

- 1 cup 1% low-fat milk
- ½ cup old-fashioned rolled oats
- 3 dried prunes, chopped
- 1 banana, diced
- 1 tablespoon crystallized ginger, chopped

1. Combine milk and oats in a small microwave-safe bowl. Microwave at HIGH 3–5 minutes.

2. Combine prunes, banana, and crystallized ginger; sprinkle over oatmeal.

Serving size: 1½ cups | Calories 420; Fat 6g (sat 2g, mono 1.5g, poly 1g); Cholesterol 10mg; Protein 15g; Carbohydrate 83g; Sugars 35g; Fiber 8g; RS 5.2g; Sodium 115mg

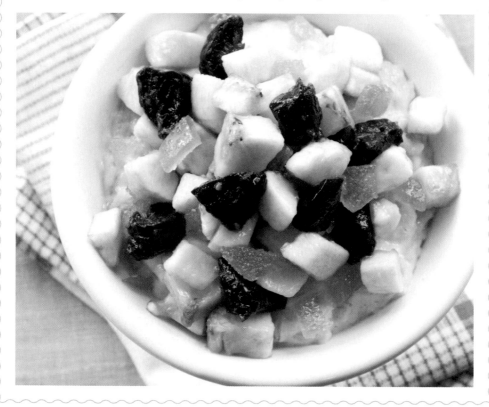

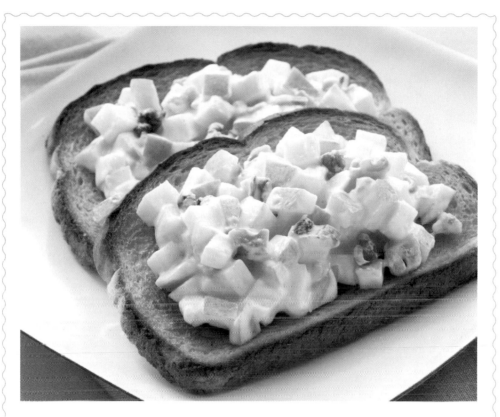

Toast with Walnut & Pear Breakfast Spread

Cottage cheese packs CLA, walnuts add some omega-3s, and pear contributes fiber, making this easy dish a great way to jump-start your metabolism in the morning.

PREP: 5 minutes
TOTAL TIME: 5 minutes
MAKES: 1 serving

Resistant Starch: **1.2** g

½ **cup low-fat, low-sodium cottage cheese**
1 **pear, chopped**
1 **tablespoon chopped walnuts**
2 **slices sourdough bread, toasted**

1. Place cottage cheese in a blender or food processor; process until smooth. Transfer to a small bowl.

2. Stir pear and walnuts into cottage cheese.

3. Spread cottage cheese mixture on toast.

Serving size: 2 pieces toast; 1 cup spread | Calories 400; Fat 7g (sat 1g, mono 1g, poly 4g); Cholesterol 5mg; Protein 22g; Carbohydrate 64g; Sugars 22g; Fiber 7g; RS 1.2g; Sodium 390mg

Polenta Fritters with Asparagus & Eggs

Asparagus is one of those vegetables that tastes wonderful when it is in season in spring, but not so much when it's out of season. During the fall and winter months, use frozen asparagus or substitute broccoli florets or spinach.

PREP: 5 minutes
COOK: 10 minutes
TOTAL TIME: 15 minutes
MAKES: 1 serving

Resistant Starch:
1.5g

Cooking spray
6 ounces polenta in tube, cut into
4 (½-inch-thick) slices
6 asparagus spears, trimmed
2 large eggs
2 tablespoons shredded Parmesan cheese
Black pepper, to taste

1. Heat a large nonstick skillet over medium heat. Coat pan with cooking spray. Add polenta and asparagus; cook 8 minutes, turning once.

2. Push polenta and asparagus to side of pan. Recoat pan with cooking spray. Add eggs, and fry until yolks are set, about 3 minutes.

3. Serve eggs on warm polenta with asparagus on the side. Sprinkle with cheese and black pepper.

Serving size: 4 pieces polenta, 2 eggs, and 6 asparagus spears | Calories 380; Fat 17g (sat 5g, mono 4g, poly 1.5g); Cholesterol 433mg; Protein 23g; Carbohydrate 30g; Sugars 6g; Fiber 4g; RS 1.5g; Sodium 600mg

★ CarbStar! ★

POLENTA

1 gram of Resistant Starch per ½ cup cooked

This soft, creamy grain is made from cooked cornmeal. Naturally high in Resistant Starch, polenta is also rich in fiber and contains a decent amount of protein, too. And it's versatile. It can be cooked into a creamy consistency or baked into crunchy sticks. In fact, you can even use it instead of white bread to make croutons.

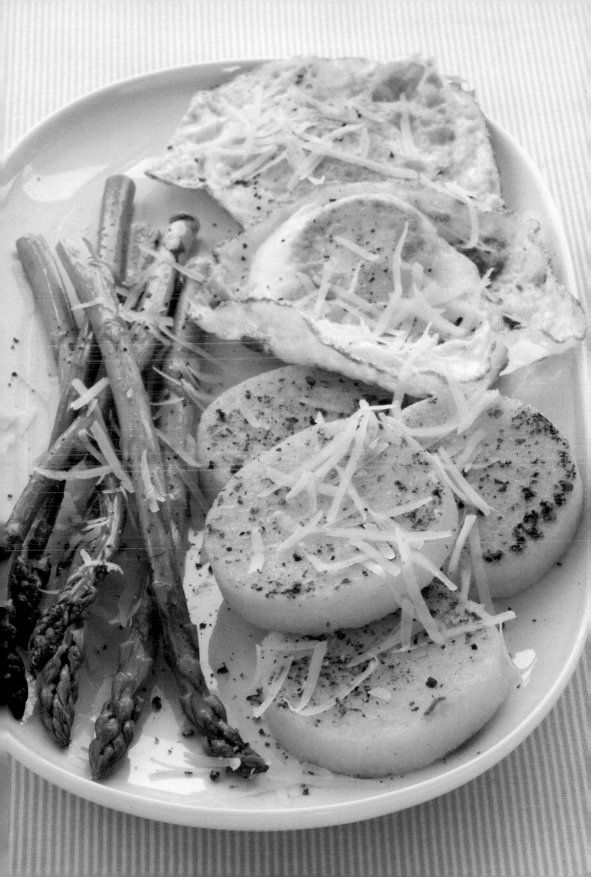

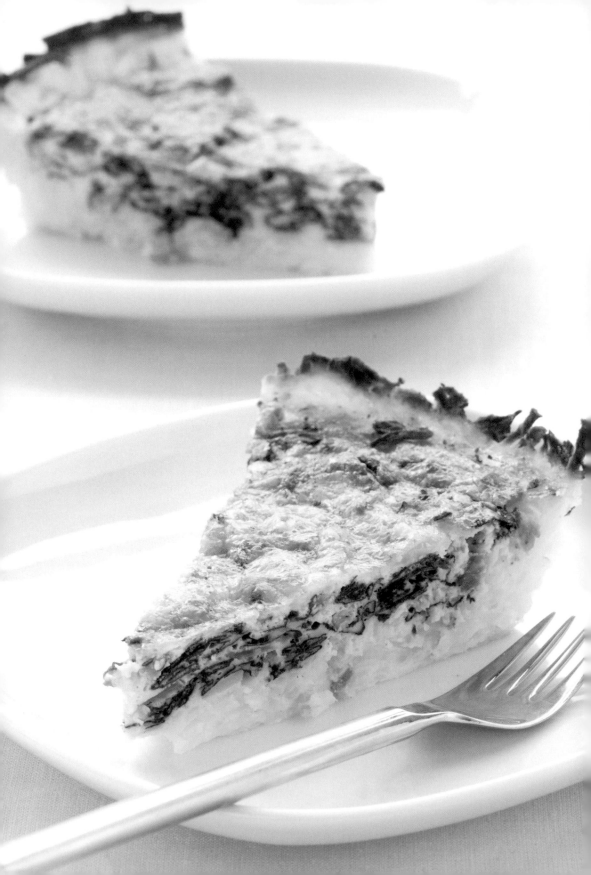

Potato-Crusted Spinach Quiche

Usually quiche crust is made from butter and flour. This version uses shredded potatoes, which cuts fat and calories and ups the amount of Resistant Starch.

PREP: 20 minutes
COOK: 1 hour
TOTAL TIME: 1 hour 20 minutes
MAKES: 4 servings

Resistant Starch:
1.4 g

- 1 tablespoon olive oil, divided
- 1 (20-ounce) package refrigerated shredded potatoes (about 3½ cups)
- 1 large egg white, whisked
- 1 tablespoon all-purpose flour
- ½ teaspoon salt
- 6 ounces fresh spinach
- ¼ cup chopped onion
- 2 tablespoons water
- 6 large eggs
- ¼ cup part-skim ricotta cheese
- ¼ teaspoon freshly ground black pepper
- 2 ounces Swiss cheese, shredded (about ½ cup)
- 1 ounce Canadian bacon, finely chopped

1. Preheat oven to 400°. Coat inside of a 9-inch deep-dish pie plate with 1 teaspoon olive oil; set aside.

2. Combine potatoes and egg white in a large bowl; toss lightly. Add flour and salt; toss to coat. Transfer to pie plate, and pat evenly into bottom and sides to form crust. Drizzle remaining 2 teaspoons oil over crust. Bake at 400° for 15 minutes or until edges begin to brown. Remove from oven. Reduce oven temperature to 350°.

3. While crust bakes, place spinach, onion, and 2 tablespoons water in a microwave-safe bowl. Microwave at HIGH 2 minutes or until spinach begins to wilt; drain. Place spinach mixture in a colander, and squeeze to drain; coarsely chop, and set aside.

4. Combine eggs and ricotta cheese in a large mixing bowl; stir with a whisk until smooth. Add black pepper. Stir in spinach mixture, half of Swiss cheese, and bacon.

5. Pour egg mixture over potato crust; spread with the back of a spoon to distribute evenly, leaving a ½-inch crust along the outer edge. Sprinkle remaining Swiss cheese on top. Bake at 350° for 50–55 minutes, until puffed and golden. Cool on a wire rack 10–15 minutes before serving. Slice into 4 equal pieces and serve.

Serving size: ¼ of quiche | Calories 380; Fat 17g (sat 6g, mono 7g, poly 2g); Cholesterol 340mg; Protein 20g; Carbohydrate 37g; Sugars 1g; Fiber 6g; RS 1.4g; Sodium 720mg

Sharp Cheddar & Egg on Rye

The protein and fiber in this easy dish will keep you satisfied all morning. If you don't like Cheddar, substitute any hard cheese.

PREP: 5 minutes
COOK: 5 minutes
TOTAL TIME: 10 minutes
MAKES: 1 serving

Cooking spray
1 **large egg**
2 **slices rye bread, toasted**
1 **slice sharp Cheddar cheese**
1 **small apple, cored and sliced**

1. Heat a nonstick skillet over medium heat. Coat pan with cooking spray. Add egg; cook until set, about 3 minutes.

2. Top toast with cheese; place egg over cheese. Serve with apple slices on the side.

Serving size: 1 sandwich and 1 apple | Calories 420; Fat 18g (sat 8g, mono 5g, poly 1.5g); Cholesterol 240mg; Protein 19g; Carbohydrate 49g; Sugars 18g; Fiber 7g; RS 1.8g; Sodium 620mg

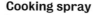

★ **CarbStar!** ★

RYE, PUMPERNICKEL, OR SOURDOUGH BREAD

0.6 to 1.3 grams of Resistant Starch per slice

Bread made from rye, pumpernickel, or sourdough is rich in Resistant Starch and fiber. One Swedish study found that rye bread decreased hunger more than whole-wheat bread.

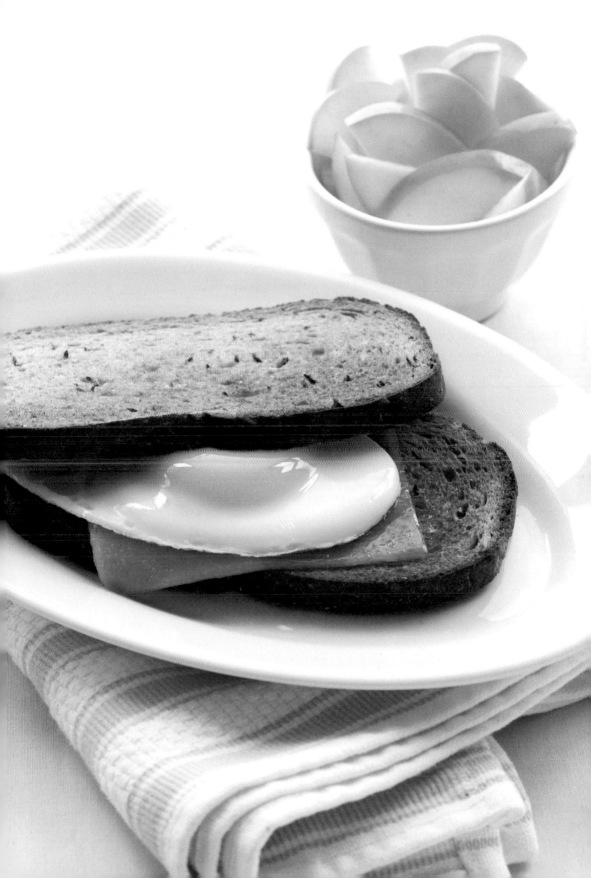

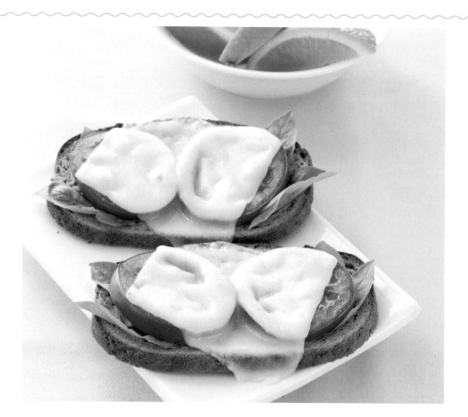

Tomato & Mozzarella Melt

This is a great breakfast idea if you prefer savory morning fare. Think of it as a mini pizza!

PREP: 5 minutes
COOK: 5 minutes
TOTAL TIME: 10 minutes
MAKES: 1 serving

2 **slices rye bread**
8 **fresh basil leaves**
4 **tomato slices**
2 **(1-ounce) slices part-skim mozzarella**
1 **orange, cut into wedges**

1. Top each bread slice with 4 basil leaves, 2 tomato slices, and 1 slice cheese.

2. Melt open-faced sandwiches in toaster oven or under broiler 4–5 minutes or until cheese is bubbling. Serve with orange wedges.

Serving size: 2 pieces topped toast and 1 orange | Calories 370; Fat 11g (sat 6g, mono 3.5g, poly 1g); Cholesterol 35mg; Protein 21g; Carbohydrate 48g; Sugars 17g; Fiber 7g; RS 1.8g; Sodium 730mg

Zucchini & Potato Scramble with Bacon

You'll be amazed how much turkey bacon tastes like the real thing for a fraction of the fat and calories. To save time on this dish, use preshredded potatoes.

PREP: 10 minutes
COOK: 15 minutes
TOTAL TIME: 25 minutes
MAKES: 1 serving

Resistant Starch:
1.4 g

1 **small potato, grated (or 1½ cups refrigerated shredded potato)**
½ **zucchini, diced**
½ **teaspoon dried oregano**
⅛ **teaspoon salt**
⅛ **teaspoon pepper**
  Cooking spray
2 **large eggs, whisked**
  Salt and pepper, to taste (optional)
2 **slices cooked turkey bacon**

1. Squeeze grated potato dry with a paper towel. Combine potato, zucchini, oregano, salt, and pepper.

2. Heat a large nonstick skillet over medium heat. Coat pan with cooking spray. Add potato mixture, and cook 10 minutes, stirring once, until tender and lightly golden. Add eggs, and cook 3–4 minutes or until eggs are set. Season to taste, and serve with bacon.

Serving size: 2 cups scramble and 2 slices turkey bacon |
Calories 370; Fat 19g (sat 4.5g, mono 6g, poly 3g); Cholesterol 450mg; Protein 21g; Carbohydrate 32g; Sugars 5g; Fiber 5g; RS 1.4g; Sodium 504mg

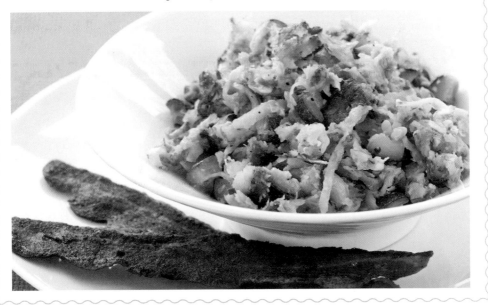

CarbLovers Immersion Lunch Recipes

Arugula Salad with Lemon-Dijon Dressing

Most croutons are made from stale white bread, which has hardly any Resistant Starch or fiber. Here, you'll use rye bread for an extra dose of Resistant Starch.

Resistant Starch: 1.8 g

PREP: 7 minutes
TOTAL TIME: 7 minutes
MAKES: 1 serving

1 tablespoon lemon juice
1 teaspoon olive oil
1 teaspoon Dijon mustard
3 cups arugula
½ cup grape tomatoes
½ cup canned white beans, rinsed and drained
2 slices rye bread, toasted and cut into 1-inch cubes
1 tablespoon shredded Parmesan cheese

1. Combine first 3 ingredients (through mustard) in a small bowl, stirring with a whisk.

2. Combine arugula, tomatoes, and beans in a large bowl. Add dressing; toss gently.

3. Top with rye bread croutons and cheese.

Serving size: 5 cups | Calories 400; Fat 10g (sat 2g, mono 4g, poly 1.5g); Cholesterol 5mg; Protein 18g; Carbohydrate 61g; Sugars 7g; Fiber 11g; RS 1.8g; Sodium 710mg

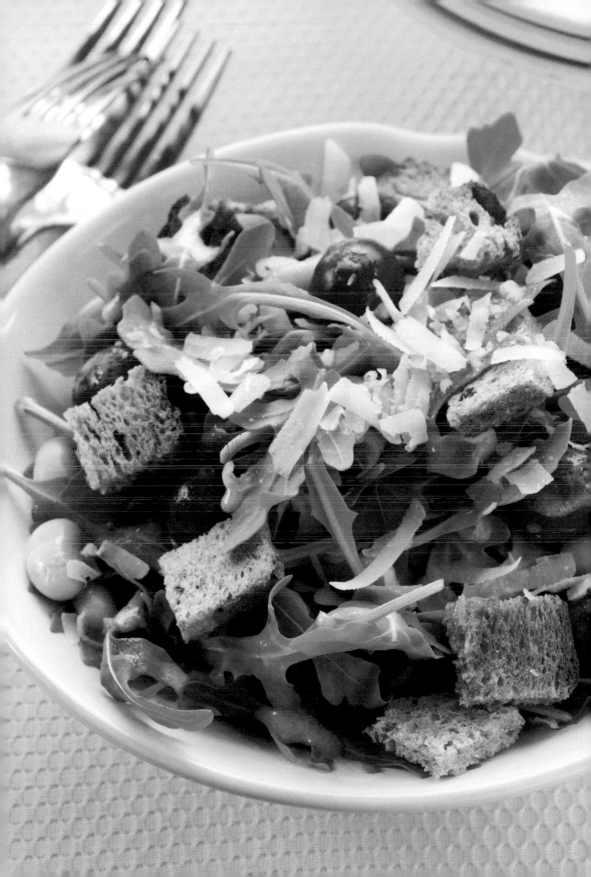

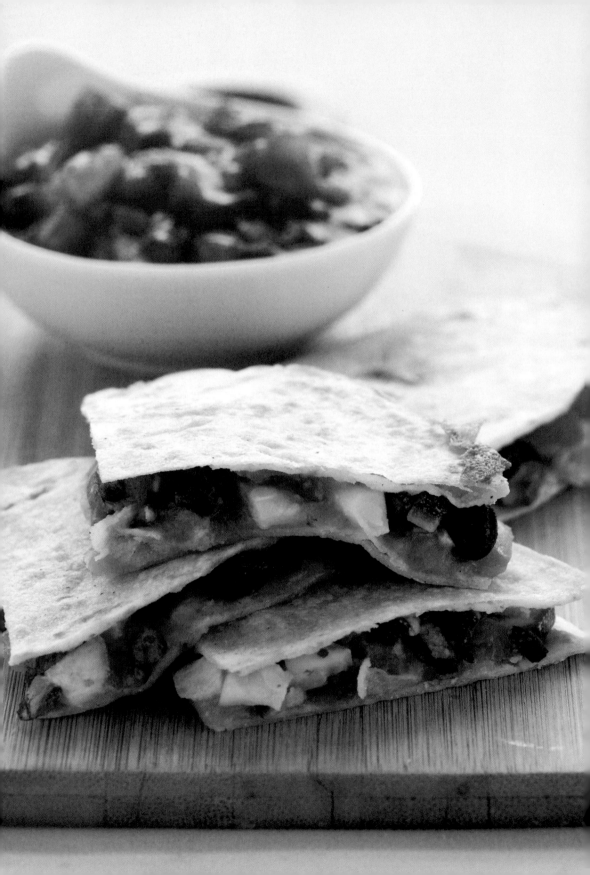

Black Bean & Zucchini Quesadillas

If you're making this lunch ahead and taking it to the office, just pop it in the microwave for 1 minute to reheat it.

PREP: 5 minutes
COOK: 2 minutes
TOTAL TIME: 7 minutes
MAKES: 1 serving

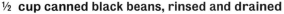

Resistant Starch: 4.7g

- ½ **cup canned black beans, rinsed and drained**
- 2 **tablespoons salsa**
- ½ **cup finely chopped zucchini**
- 4 **(6-inch) corn tortillas**
- 4 **tablespoons shredded Cheddar cheese**

1. Combine beans and salsa in a small bowl; mash with a fork. Stir in zucchini.

2. Layer 2 tortillas with half of the bean mixture, sprinkle with 2 tablespoons cheese, and top with remaining 2 tortillas. Repeat with remaining tortillas, bean mixture, and cheese.

3. In broiler or toaster oven, cook quesadillas 1 minute on each side until cheese is melted and bubbly.

Serving size: 2 quesadillas | Calories 400; Fat 11g (sat 6g, mono 0.5g, poly 1.5g); Cholesterol 30mg; Protein 18g; Carbohydrate 65g; Sugars 4g; Fiber 13g; RS 4.7g; Sodium 670mg

Curried Egg Salad Sandwich

The curry adds a health-promoting antioxidant jolt to this traditional comfort dish. To save prep time, batch-cook a dozen eggs at the beginning of each week so you always have some handy.

PREP: 7 minutes
TOTAL TIME: 7 minutes
MAKES: 1 serving

Resistant Starch:
1.8 g

 2 **hard-cooked eggs, chopped**
 2 **tablespoons plain low-fat Greek yogurt**
 2 **tablespoons chopped red bell pepper**
 ¼ **teaspoon curry powder**
     Dash of salt
 ⅛ **teaspoon pepper**
 2 **slices rye bread, toasted**
 ½ **cup fresh spinach**
 1 **orange, sliced**

1. Combine eggs, yogurt, bell pepper, curry powder, salt, and pepper in a small bowl; stir well.

2. Place spinach on 1 slice of bread, and top with egg salad. Place other piece of bread on top. Slice in half on the diagonal with a sharp knife. Serve with orange slices.

Serving size: 1 sandwich and 1 orange | Calories 414; Fat 14g (sat 4g, mono 5g, poly 2g); Cholesterol 426mg; Protein 22g; Carbohydrate 51g; Sugars 18g; Fiber 8g; RS 1.8g; Sodium 654mg

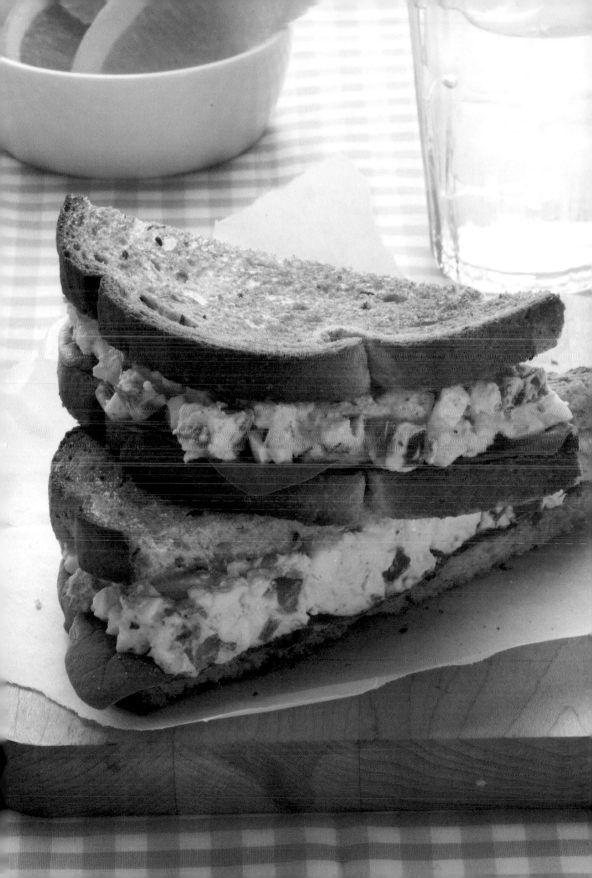

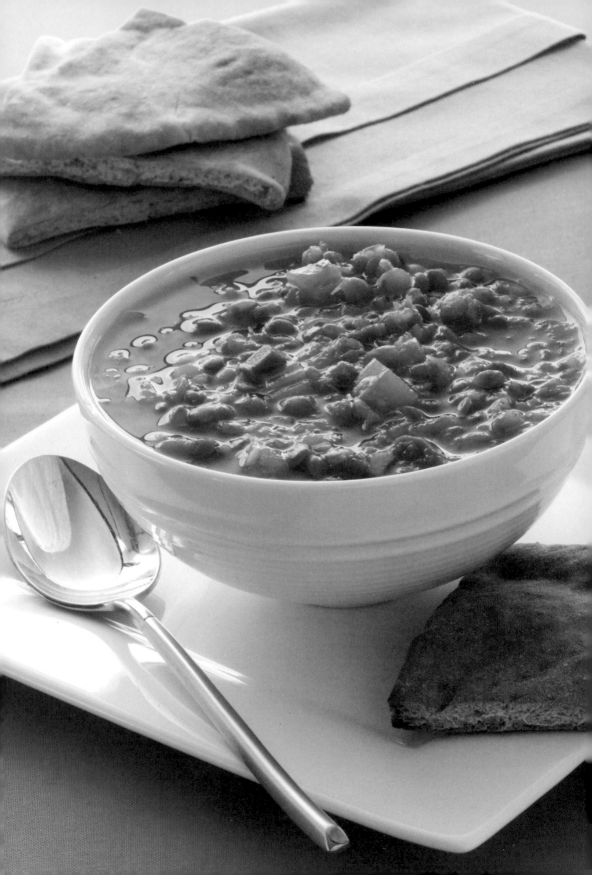

Greek Lentil Soup with Toasted Pita

Lentils are a great source of Resistant Starch and fiber. Double or triple this recipe, and freeze leftovers in individual containers.

PREP: 10 minutes
COOK: 20 minutes
TOTAL TIME: 30 minutes
MAKES: 4 servings

Resistant Starch:
1.9g

- 1 **tablespoon olive oil**
- 2 **celery stalks, chopped**
- 2 **carrots, peeled and chopped**
- 1 **onion, chopped**
- 2 **garlic cloves, minced**
- 2 **teaspoons dried oregano**
- ½ **teaspoon salt**
- ½ **teaspoon pepper**
- 8 **cups water**
- 1 **cup dry lentils**
- 2 **tablespoons fresh lemon juice (about 1 lemon)**
- 4 **whole-grain pitas, each cut into 4 triangles and toasted**

1. Heat oil in a large Dutch oven over medium heat. Add celery, carrot, onion, garlic, oregano, salt, and pepper; cook 5 minutes.

2. Add 8 cups water and lentils. Simmer, partially covered, 15 minutes.

3. With a hand blender or potato masher, puree soup until semismooth and thick.

4. Drizzle with lemon juice; serve with toasted pita.

Serving size: 2 cups soup and 1 pita | Calories 370; Fat 6g (sat 0.5g, mono 2.5g, poly 1.5g); Cholesterol 0mg; Protein 19g; Carbohydrate 65g; Sugars 6g; Fiber 21g; RS 1.9g; Sodium 680mg

Ham, Sliced Pear & Swiss Sandwich

The pear adds flavor, texture, and fiber to this traditional ham-and-Swiss sandwich.

PREP: 10 minutes
TOTAL TIME: 10 minutes
MAKES: 1 serving

Resistant Starch: **2.6** g

- 1 tablespoon plain low-fat Greek yogurt
- ¼ teaspoon dried dill
- 2 slices pumpernickel bread
- 1 (1-ounce) slice lean ham
- 1 small pear, thinly sliced
- 1 (1-ounce) slice low-sodium Swiss cheese

1. Combine yogurt and dill in a small bowl; stir until blended.

2. Spread yogurt mixture on 1 slice of bread. Top with ham, half of the pear slices, cheese, and remaining bread slice. Slice in half using a sharp knife. Serve with remaining pear slices on the side.

Serving size: 1 sandwich and 1 pear | Calories 410; Fat 13g (sat 6g, mono 4g, poly 1g); Cholesterol 43mg; Protein 22g; Carbohydrate 55g; Sugars 16g; Fiber 9g; RS 2.6g; Sodium 710mg

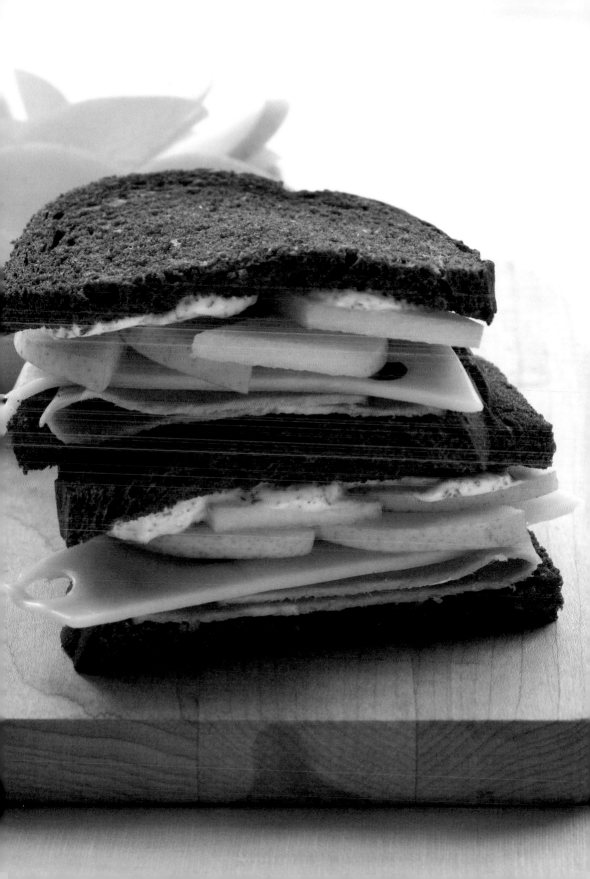

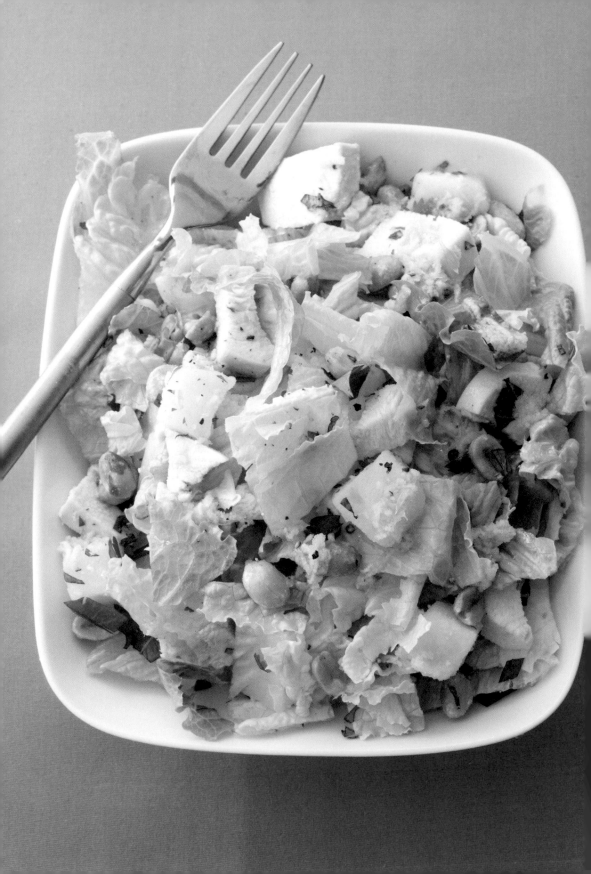

Indian Chicken Salad with Peanuts

If you are short on time, use precooked white meat chicken strips or rotisserie chicken and bottled light sesame-ginger dressing for this recipe.

PREP: 10 minutes
COOK: 5 minutes
TOTAL TIME: 15 minutes
MAKES: 1 serving

Resistant Starch:

2 g

- 1 **cup potato, cut into ½-inch cubes**
  Cooking spray
- ⅛ **teaspoon salt**
- ⅛ **teaspoon pepper**
- 2 **tablespoons water**
- 2 **tablespoons lime juice**
- 1 **teaspoon dark sesame oil**
- 1 **teaspoon honey**
- 1 **teaspoon grated peeled fresh ginger**
- 3 **cups chopped Romaine lettuce**
- ¼ **cup (2 ounces) grilled or baked skinless chicken, chopped**
- 2 **tablespoons chopped peanuts**
- 1 **tablespoon chopped fresh mint**
- 1 **tablespoon chopped fresh cilantro**

1. Place potato in a microwave-safe dish. Spray potato with cooking spray, and sprinkle with salt and pepper. Add 2 tablespoons water; cover and microwave at HIGH 5 minutes or until tender.

2. Combine lime juice, oil, honey, and ginger in a small bowl; stir well with a whisk.

3. Combine potato, lettuce, chicken, peanuts, mint, and cilantro in a large bowl. Add dressing; toss gently to coat.

Serving size: 4½ cups | Calories 420, Fat 17g (sat 2.5g, mono 7g, poly 6g); Cholesterol 50mg; Protein 27g; Carbohydrate 44g; Sugars 10g; Fiber 8g; RS 2g; Sodium 360mg

Mediterranean Pasta Salad

Peas are an easy way to bump up the Resistant Starch in any dish. Just keep a bag of frozen peas in the freezer so you can easily add them to this and other grain salads.

PREP: 15 minutes
COOK: 15 minutes
TOTAL TIME: 30 minutes
MAKES: 4 servings

Resistant Starch: **2.4**g

- 1 cup uncooked multigrain farfalle (bow tie pasta)
- 1 teaspoon lemon zest
- 2 tablespoons lemon juice
- 2 teaspoons olive oil
- 1 (14-ounce) can artichoke hearts packed in water, drained and chopped
- 1 cup fresh part-skim mozzarella cheese, cubed
- ¼ cup chopped bottled roasted red bell pepper
- ¼ cup chopped fresh parsley
- ½ cup frozen peas

1. Cook pasta according to package instructions, omitting salt and fat.

2. While pasta cooks, combine zest and juice of 1 lemon and 2 teaspoons olive oil in a large bowl; stir well with a whisk. Add artichoke hearts, cheese, bell pepper, and parsley; toss to combine.

3. Place the peas in a colander; when the pasta is cooked, drain pasta over peas. Shake well to drain, but do not run under cold water. Add the pasta and peas to the artichoke mixture, and toss well until thoroughly combined. Serve warm or at room temperature.

Serving size: 2 cups | Calories 418; Fat 16g (sat 8g, mono 2g, poly 1g); Cholesterol 45mg; Protein 20g; Carbohydrate 50g; Sugars 3g; Fiber 8g; RS 2.4g; Sodium 196mg

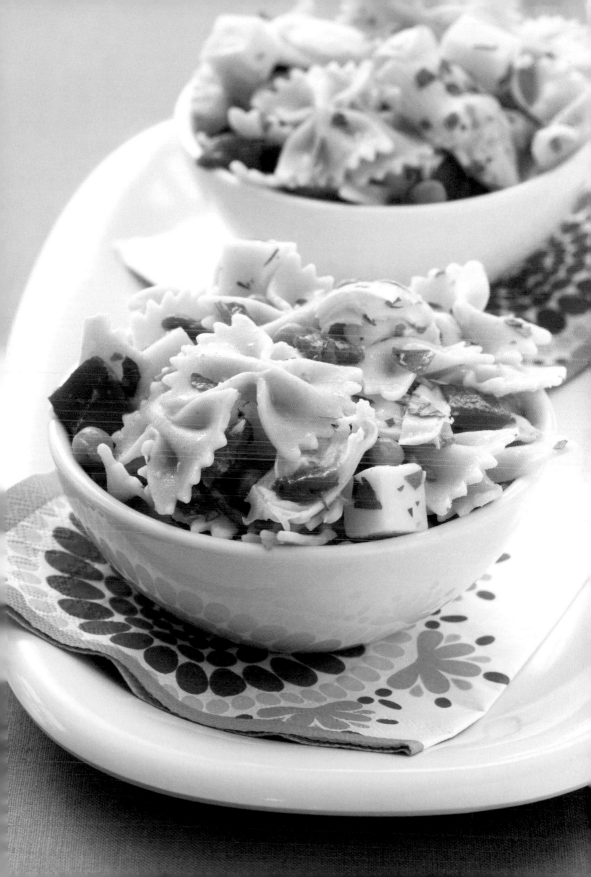

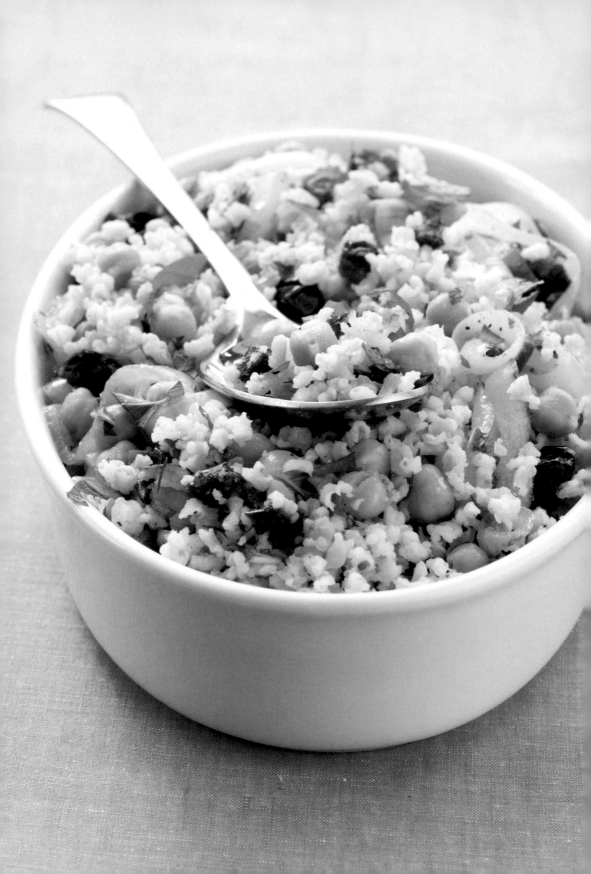

Middle Eastern Rice Salad

Resistant Starch:
4.1 g

The dates in this recipe provide plenty of appetite-suppressing fiber, while the brown rice and chickpeas pack more than 4 grams of Resistant Starch per serving.

PREP: 15 minutes
COOK: 5 minutes
TOTAL TIME: 20 minutes
MAKES: 4 servings

- 2 **tablespoons olive oil**
- ½ **Vidalia or other sweet onion, thinly sliced (about ¾ cup)**
- 1 **(16-ounce) can chickpeas, rinsed and drained**
- ½ **teaspoon ground cumin**
- ¼ **teaspoon salt**
  Freshly ground black pepper, to taste
- 3 **cups cooked brown rice**
- ½ **cup chopped dates**
- ¼ **cup chopped fresh mint**
- ¼ **cup chopped fresh parsley**

1. Heat oil in a large nonstick skillet over medium-high heat. Add onion, and cook, stirring often, 5 minutes or until onion begins to brown. Remove from heat, and stir in chickpeas, cumin, and salt. Season to taste with freshly ground black pepper.

2. Combine rice, onion-and-chickpea mixture, dates, mint, and parsley in a large bowl. Toss well until thoroughly combined. Serve warm or at room temperature.

Serving size: 1¼ cups | Calories 380; Fat 9g (sat 1g, mono 5.5g, poly 1g); Cholesterol 0mg; Protein 8g; Carbohydrate 67g; Sugars 18g; Fiber 8g; RS 4.1g; Sodium 360mg

★ CarbStar! ★
BROWN RICE
1.7 grams of Resistant Starch per ½ cup

Brown rice may cook more slowly than its refined white cousins, but it digests more slowly, too. One study found that blood sugar levels were 24 percent lower in people who consumed brown rice, compared with participants in a control group. Another study found that eating a black and brown rice mix is healthier than eating white rice; it resulted in a greater reduction in weight, body mass index, and body fat.

Moroccan Chicken Pita

This quick-and-easy lunch option can be made even easier if you use precooked chicken strips or rotisserie chicken.

PREP: 10 minutes
TOTAL TIME: 10 minutes
MAKES: 1 serving

Resistant Starch:

1g

- 4 tablespoons plain low-fat Greek yogurt
- ½ teaspoon honey
- ⅛ teaspoon salt
- ⅛ teaspoon ground cumin
- ⅛ teaspoon ground cinnamon
- ⅓ cup (3 ounces) grilled or baked chicken, chopped
- ½ cup shredded carrot
- 2 tablespoons chopped dates
- 1 whole-grain pita, halved
- ½ cup fresh spinach

1. Combine first 5 ingredients (through cinnamon) in a small bowl, stirring well with a whisk.

2. Combine chicken, carrot, and dates in a bowl. Add dressing; toss gently to coat.

3. Fill pita halves with chicken mixture and spinach.

Serving size: 2 stuffed pita halves | Calories 420; Fat 6g (sat 1.5, mono 1g, poly 1.5g); Cholesterol 75mg; Protein 39g; Carbohydrate 56g; Sugars 24g; Fiber 8g; RS 1g; Sodium 750mg

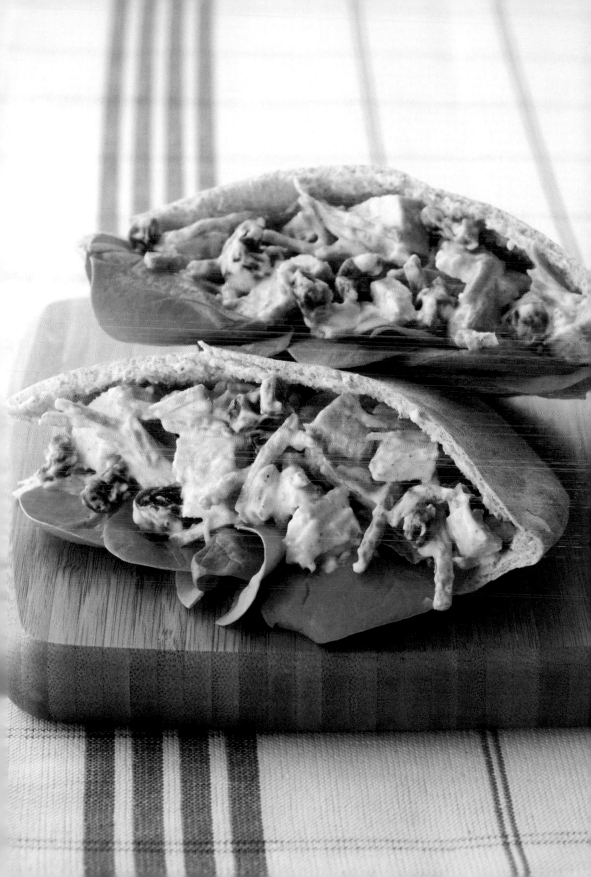

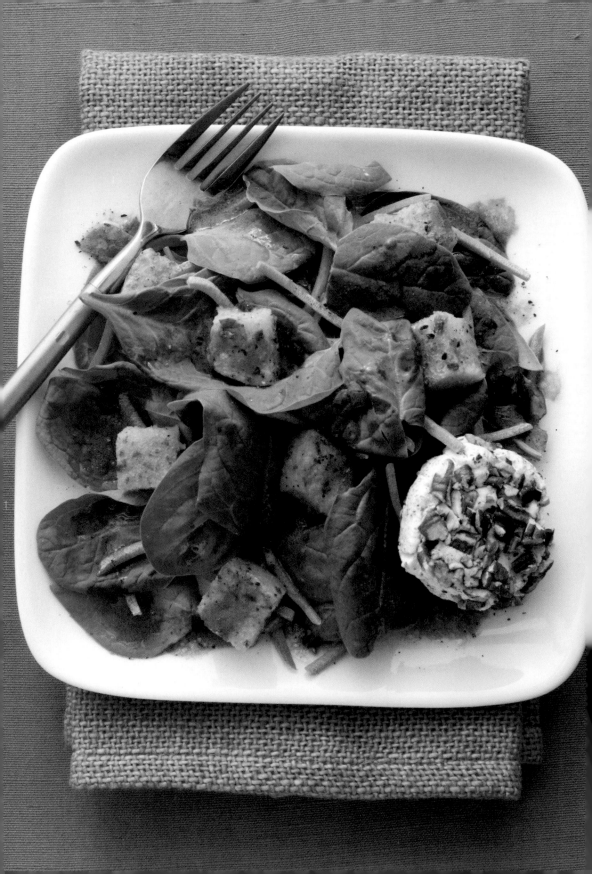

Pecan-Crusted Goat Cheese Salad
with Pomegranate Vinaigrette

Resistant Starch:

1g

Rich in MUFAs, CLA, fiber, and oleic acid, this just might win the award for the most filling, slimming, and satisfying salad ever created.

PREP: 5 minutes
COOK: 10 minutes
TOTAL TIME: 15 minutes

¼ **tube of polenta (4 ounces), cut into 1-inch cubes**
  Cooking spray
1 **ounce goat cheese**
1 **tablespoon chopped pecans**
2 **tablespoons pomegranate juice**
1 **teaspoon olive oil**
1 **teaspoon Dijon mustard**
3 **cups fresh spinach**
½ **cup shredded carrot**

1. Heat a large nonstick skillet over medium heat. Coat polenta cubes with cooking spray. Add to pan, and cook 5 minutes. Turn croutons; cook 5 minutes more or until golden.

2. Shape goat cheese into a patty; coat with chopped pecans.

3. Combine juice, oil, and mustard in a small bowl; stir well with a whisk.

4. Arrange spinach and carrot on a plate. Top with polenta cubes, pecan-crusted goat cheese, and dressing.

Serving size: 4½ cups | Calories 370; Fat 21g (sat 7g, mono 8g, poly 2g); Cholesterol 20mg; Protein 11g; Carbohydrate 36g; Sugars 10g; Fiber 7g; RS 1g; Sodium 720mg

Pesto Turkey Club

Pesto packs two metabolism boosters—olive oil and pine nuts. Add that to the pumpernickel bread (Resistant Starch), apple (fiber), and turkey (protein), and you've got an ultraslimming club sandwich.

Resistant Starch:

2.6g

PREP: 5 minutes
TOTAL TIME: 5 minutes
MAKES: 1 serving

- 2 **teaspoons prepared pesto**
- 2 **slices pumpernickel bread**
- 1 **(1-ounce) slice turkey**
- 1 **low-sodium turkey-bacon slice, cooked**
- 2 **Romaine lettuce leaves**
- 4 **slices tomato**
- 1 **apple**

1. Spread pesto on 1 slice of bread. Top with turkey, bacon, lettuce, tomato, and remaining bread slice. Cut sandwich in half using a sharp knife.

2. Serve sandwich with apple.

Serving size: 1 sandwich and 1 apple | Calories 390; Fat 11g (sat 3g, mono 4g, poly 1g); Cholesterol 32mg; Protein 20g; Carbohydrate 60g; Sugars 23g; Fiber 10g; RS 2.6g; Sodium 614mg

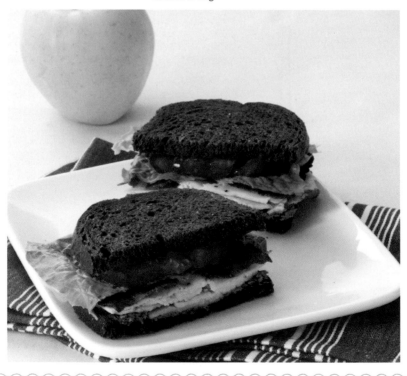

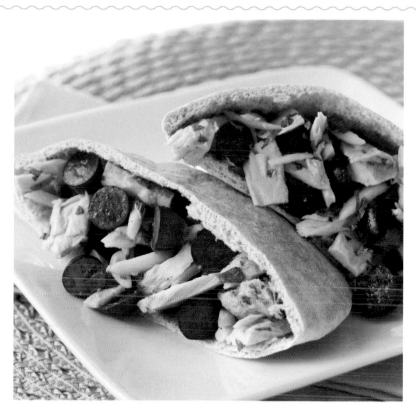

Red Grape & Tuna Salad Pita

Tuna is a rich source of metabolism-boosting omega-3 fatty acids. Add that to the MUFAs in the almonds and the Resistant Starch in the pita, and you've tripled the boost to your metabolism.

PREP: 7 minutes
TOTAL TIME: 7 minutes
MAKES: 1 serving

½ **can (3 ounces) tuna in water, drained**
½ **cup red grapes, halved**
1 **tablespoon slivered almonds**
1 **tablespoon chopped fresh mint**
1 **tablespoon lemon juice**
2 **teaspoons olive oil**
⅛ **teaspoon black pepper**
1 **whole-grain pita, halved**

1. Combine first 7 ingredients (through pepper) in a small bowl. Toss gently. Serve in pita halves.

Serving size: 2 stuffed pita halves | Calories 410; Fat 15g (sat 1.5g, mono 9g, poly 3g); Cholesterol 45mg; Protein 28g; Carbohydrate 45g; Sugars 14g; Fiber 6g; RS 1g; Sodium 700mg

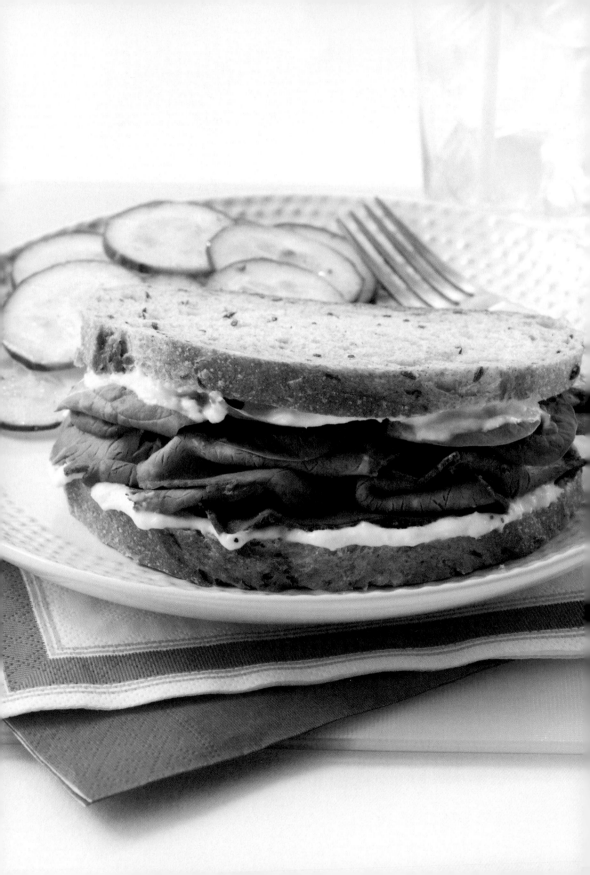

Roast Beef Sandwich with Horseradish Aioli

The rye bread in this sandwich packs a good amount of Resistant Starch, and the veggies have plenty of fiber to keep you feeling satisfied all afternoon long.

PREP: 7 minutes
TOTAL TIME: 7 minutes
MAKES: 1 serving

Resistant Starch: **1.8** g

- 2 **tablespoons reduced-fat mayonnaise**
- 2 **teaspoons prepared horseradish**
- 2 **slices rye bread**
- 2 **(1-ounce) slices roast beef**
- ½ **cup fresh spinach**
- 1 **cup sliced cucumbers**
- 1 **tablespoon less-sodium, low-fat Italian dressing**

1. Combine mayonnaise and horseradish in a small bowl; stir well with a whisk.

2. Spread mayonnaise mixture on both bread slices. Top 1 bread slice with roast beef, spinach, and remaining bread slice.

3. Serve with cucumber slices drizzled with dressing.

Serving size: 1 sandwich and 1 cup cucumber salad | Calories 350; Fat 10g (sat 2g, mono 3g, poly 4g); Cholesterol 38mg; Protein 24g; Carbohydrate 43g; Sugars 6g; Fiber 5g; RS 1.8g; Sodium 546mg

Smoked Salmon & Avocado Hand Rolls

There's no raw seafood in this roll, so even those who avoid sushi for that reason can enjoy this. To save time, use the brown rice that you batch-cooked earlier in the week, or use a precooked variety.

PREP: 10 minutes
TOTAL TIME: 10 minutes
MAKES: 1 serving

Resistant Starch:
2.6g

- ¼ **avocado, mashed**
- 3 **nori (seaweed) sheets**
- ¾ **cup cooked and cooled brown rice**
- 1 **(1-ounce) slice smoked salmon**
- 3 **tomato slices**
- 3 **tablespoons chopped red onion**
- 1 **tablespoon capers**

1. Spread avocado on nori sheets.

2. Top the avocado with brown rice, salmon, tomato, onion, and capers; roll up the nori sheets. Slice rolls into pieces with a serrated knife.

Serving size: 3 rolls | Calories 400; Fat 12g (sat 2g, mono 7g, poly 2.5g); Cholesterol 45mg; Protein 26g; Carbohydrate 47g; Sugars 3g; Fiber 9g; RS 2.6g; Sodium 430mg

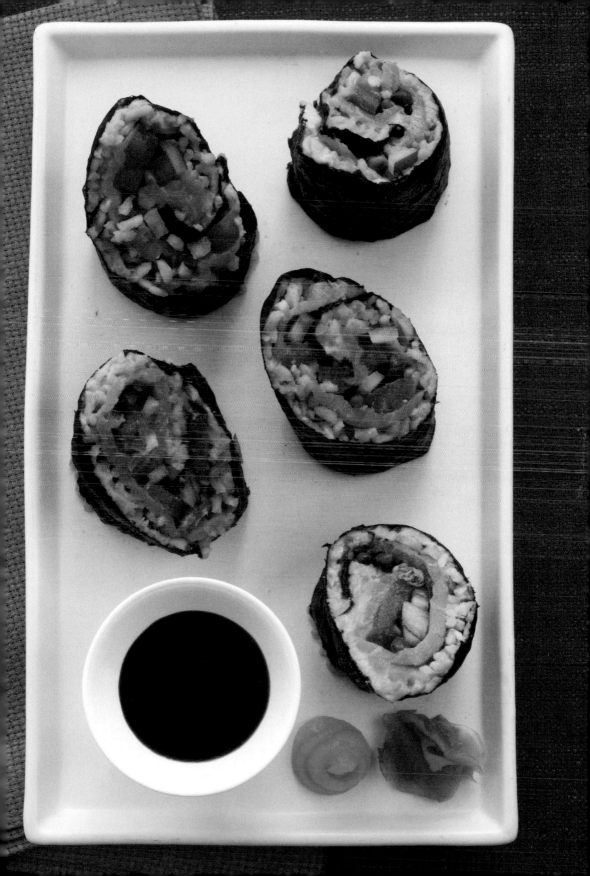

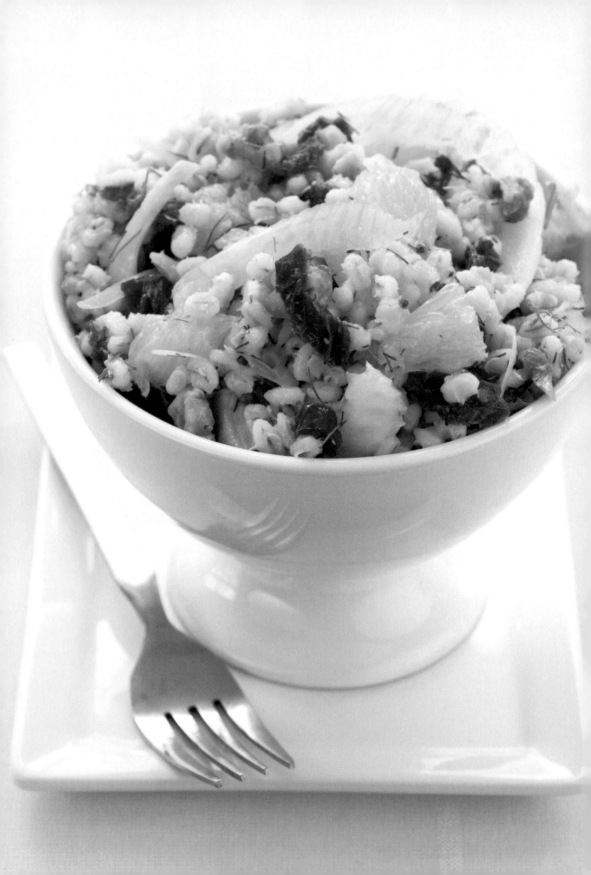

Tuscan Barley Salad

Make sure to batch-cook barley earlier in the week to speed the prep time for this high-fiber, high–Resistant Starch dish. The orange zest adds a wonderful bright flavor to the salad, which tastes even better the next day.

PREP: 20 minutes
COOK: 5 minutes
TOTAL TIME: 25 minutes
MAKES: 4 servings

Resistant Starch: **3.8**g

- ½ cup chopped walnuts
- 1 navel orange
- 2 tablespoons olive oil
- ¼ teaspoon salt
- 4 cups cooked pearl barley
- ½ pound fennel bulb, thinly sliced (about 1 cup), plus 2 tablespoons chopped fennel fronds
- ¼ cup thinly sliced sun-dried tomatoes, packed in water

1. Toast walnuts in a nonstick skillet over medium heat, stirring frequently to prevent scorching, 5 minutes or until fragrant. Transfer walnuts to a plate, and set aside.

2. Use a microplane grater or vegetable peeler to remove the zest from the orange (only the colorful skin, not the bitter white part underneath). If using a vegetable peeler, chop the zest finely; place zest in a large bowl. Carefully peel the orange with a knife, removing all of the white pith and outer membrane. Hold the fruit over the bowl and cut between the inner membranes to release the orange segments; let them drop into the bowl, along with the juices. Use clean hands to tear larger segments into smaller pieces.

3. Add olive oil and salt; toss until combined. Add barley, fennel, sun-dried tomatoes, and reserved walnuts. Toss until thoroughly combined.

Serving size: 1½ cups | Calories 380; Fat 17g (sat 2g, mono 6.5g, poly 8g); Cholesterol 0mg; Protein 7g; Carbohydrate 54g; Sugars 5g; Fiber 9g; RS 3.8g; Sodium 230mg

★ CarbStar! ★

BARLEY

1.9 grams of Resistant Starch per ½ cup

In addition to Resistant Starch, barley is rich in soluble and insoluble fiber, which reduces appetite and keeps you regular. In one University of Minnesota study, participants reported significantly less hunger before lunch after they consumed a barley snack, compared with participants who consumed a snack made of refined rice.

CarbLovers Immersion Dinner Recipes

Barley Risotto Primavera

Swapping the usual Arborio rice used in risotto for barley boosts fiber and Resistant Starch. Save prep time by batch-cooking the barley at the beginning of the week.

PREP: 15 minutes
COOK: 20 minutes
TOTAL TIME: 35 minutes
MAKES: 4 servings

Resistant Starch: 4.1g

- 2 tablespoons olive oil
- 2 carrots, peeled and chopped (about ⅔ cup)
- ½ cup finely chopped onion
- 2 garlic cloves, minced
- ½ teaspoon dried thyme
- 3 cups cooked quick-cooking barley
- ½ cup white wine (optional)
- 1½ to 2 cups low-sodium vegetable broth, divided
- 1 small zucchini, chopped (about 1 cup)
- ½ red bell pepper, chopped (about ¾ cup)
- ½ yellow bell pepper, chopped (about ¾ cup)
- ¼ teaspoon salt
  Freshly ground black pepper, to taste
- 1½ cups frozen peas
- ¾ cup grated Parmesan cheese

1. Heat oil in a large nonstick skillet over medium-high heat. Add carrot and onion, and cook 4–5 minutes until onion begins to brown. Add garlic and thyme; cook 1 minute or until fragrant.

2. Reduce heat to medium; stir in barley and white wine (if using) or ½ cup broth; cook 1 minute or until liquid is absorbed. Add zucchini, bell peppers, and ¾ cup broth; cook 4–5 minutes, stirring occasionally, until liquid is absorbed. Add remaining ¾ cup broth; cook until vegetables are tender and most of liquid has been absorbed. Add ¼ teaspoon salt and freshly ground black pepper.

3. Stir in peas; remove from heat. Let stand 1–2 minutes or until peas are thawed but still bright green. Stir in Parmesan cheese just before serving.

Serving size: 1¾ cups | Calories 380; Fat 14g (sat 4g, mono 5g, poly 1g); Cholesterol 15mg; Protein 16g; Carbohydrate 50g; Sugars 5g; Fiber 9g; RS 4.1g; Sodium 620mg

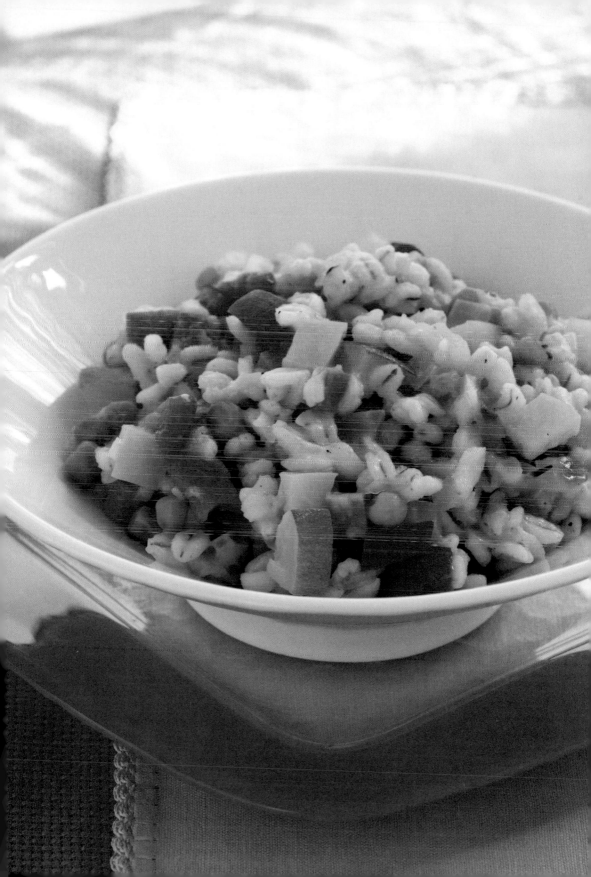

Bistro-Style Sirloin with New Potatoes

Here's a classic, high-protein meal. Boiling the potatoes whole kicks the Resistant Starch factor up several notches.

PREP: 10 minutes
COOK: 25 minutes
TOTAL TIME: 35 minutes
MAKES: 4 servings

Resistant Starch:

2.3 g

1½ **pounds new potatoes**
1¼ **pounds lean sirloin, trimmed of visible fat**
½ **teaspoon salt, divided**
  Freshly ground black pepper, to taste
6 **teaspoons olive oil, divided**
1 **large shallot, finely chopped (about 3 tablespoons)**
½ **cup dry red wine**
4 **cups arugula, divided**

1. Place potatoes in a large saucepan; cover with cold water. Bring water to a boil, and cook 15 minutes or until potatoes can be pierced with a fork. Drain and cool potatoes. Slice potatoes in half.

2. While potatoes cook, divide steak into 4 equal portions, and sprinkle with ¼ teaspoon salt and freshly ground black pepper. Heat 2 teaspoons oil in a large heavy skillet over medium-high heat. Add steaks to pan, and cook 4–6 minutes per side or until a meat thermometer inserted into thickest part of the steak reads 160°. Transfer steaks to a plate, and keep warm.

3. Reduce heat to medium-low; add 2 teaspoons oil and shallot to pan. Arrange potatoes, cut sides down, in pan, and cook 5 minutes or until potatoes begin to brown.

4. Season with remaining ¼ teaspoon salt and freshly ground black pepper. Transfer potatoes to a bowl, and keep warm.

5. Increase heat to medium-high. Add wine, and gently scrape pan to loosen browned bits. Add remaining 2 teaspoons olive oil, and cook until liquid is reduced by half. Place 1 cup arugula on each of 4 plates; divide steak and potatoes evenly. Top each serving with approximately 1 tablespoon sauce.

Serving size: 1 steak, 1 cup potatoes, 1 cup arugula, and 1 tablespoon sauce | Calories 400; Fat 13g (sat 3g, mono 7g, poly 1g); Cholesterol 60mg; Protein 35g; Carbohydrate 30g; Sugars 3g; Fiber 4g; RS 2.3g; Sodium 390mg

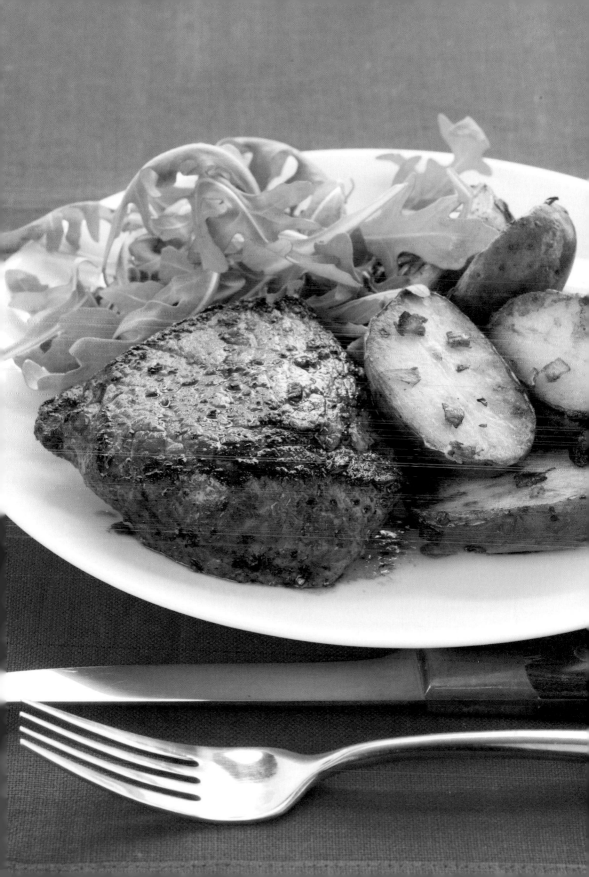

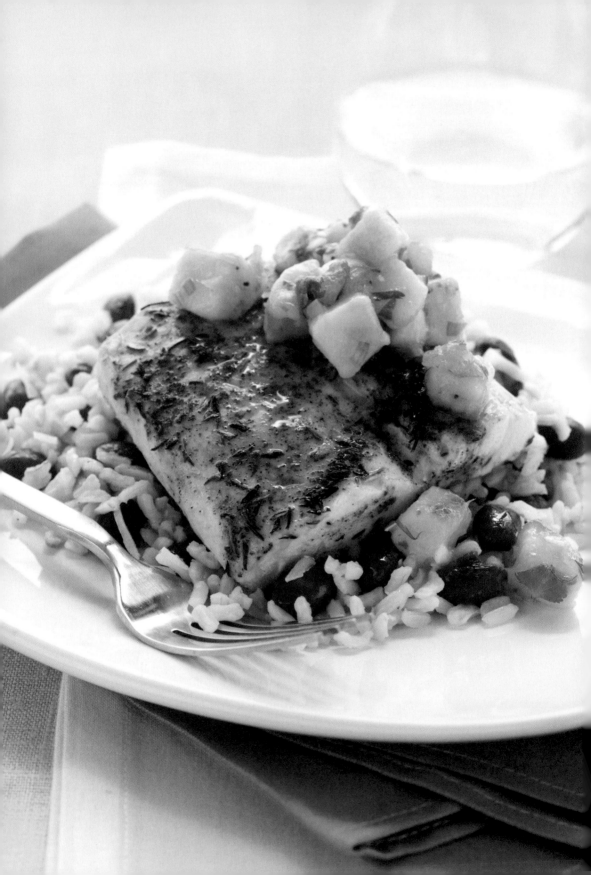

Caribbean Mahi Mahi with Banana Chutney

Nearly every metabolism booster on *The CarbLovers Diet* is included in this recipe, with three Resistant Starch stars: brown rice, banana, and beans.

PREP: 15 minutes
BAKE: 5 minutes
TOTAL TIME: 20 minutes
MAKES: 4 servings

Resistant Starch: 4.8 g

2 cups water
2 cups uncooked quick-cooking brown rice (such as Uncle Ben's Whole Grain Boil in Bag Brown Rice; use 1 bag)
¼ cup flaked sweetened coconut
1 cup canned red beans, rinsed and drained
¼ teaspoon salt
¼ teaspoon ground allspice
¼ teaspoon dried thyme
¼ teaspoon cayenne pepper
1 pound skinless mahi mahi fillets, cut into 4 pieces
½ teaspoon olive oil
2 tablespoons mango chutney
2 bananas, peeled and chopped
1 scallion, finely chopped
1 tablespoon chopped fresh cilantro

1. Preheat broiler.

2. Bring 2 cups water to a boil in a medium saucepan over medium-high heat.

3. If using Uncle Ben's Boil in Bag, drop in bag, and boil 10 minutes; remove from bag and add coconut. Reduce heat to low. Simmer, covered, 5 minutes. Turn off heat; stir in beans, and set aside. (If using regular quick cooking brown rice, add rice and coconut to boiling water. Reduce heat to low. Simmer, covered, 5 minutes. Turn off heat; stir in beans, and set aside.)

4. While rice cooks, combine salt, allspice, thyme, and cayenne pepper in a small bowl; set aside.

5. Arrange fish on a baking sheet. Drizzle oil over fish. Sprinkle half of seasoning mixture over fish; turn fish over, and sprinkle with remaining seasoning.

6. Broil for 5–6 minutes or until fish flakes easily with a fork.

7. While fish broils, combine chutney, banana, scallions, and cilantro in a small bowl. Serve rice and bean mixture topped with fish and chutney mixture.

Serving size: 4 ounces mahi mahi, 1 cup rice and beans, and about ¼ cup chutney | Calories 410; Fat 4g (sat 2g, mono 1g, poly 0.5g); Cholesterol 85mg; Protein 29g; Carbohydrate 65g; Sugars 16g; Fiber 7g; RS 4.8g; Sodium 510mg

Fish Tacos with Sesame-Ginger Slaw

Corn tortillas add a hearty dose of Resistant Starch to this traditional Tex-Mex dish, while shredded coleslaw mix lends fiber and crunch.

PREP: 10 minutes
COOK: 10 minutes
TOTAL TIME: 20 minutes
MAKES: 4 servings

Resistant Starch:

2.4 g

- 1½ **pounds tilapia fillets**
   Cooking spray
- ¼ **teaspoon salt**
- ¼ **teaspoon pepper**
- 3 **tablespoons plain low-fat Greek yogurt**
- 2 **tablespoons lime juice**
- 1 **tablespoon dark sesame oil**
- 1 **tablespoon low-sodium soy sauce**
- 2 **teaspoons grated peeled fresh ginger**
- 1 **teaspoon honey**
- 3 **cups shredded coleslaw mix**
- 12 **(6-inch) corn tortillas, warmed**

1. Heat a nonstick skillet or grill pan over medium heat. Coat fish with cooking spray; sprinkle with salt and pepper. Add fish to pan; cook 10–12 minutes, turning once, until fish flakes easily with a fork.

2. Combine yogurt and next 5 ingredients (through honey) in a small bowl, stirring with a whisk. Combine dressing and coleslaw mix, tossing to coat.

3. Flake fish into pieces with a fork. Place 2 ounces fish in each tortilla. Top with coleslaw.

Serving size: 3 tacos | Calories 390; Fat 9g (sat 2g, mono 3g, poly 3g); Cholesterol 85mg; Protein 40g; Carbohydrate 38g; Sugars 4g; Fiber 6g; RS 2.4g; Sodium 430mg

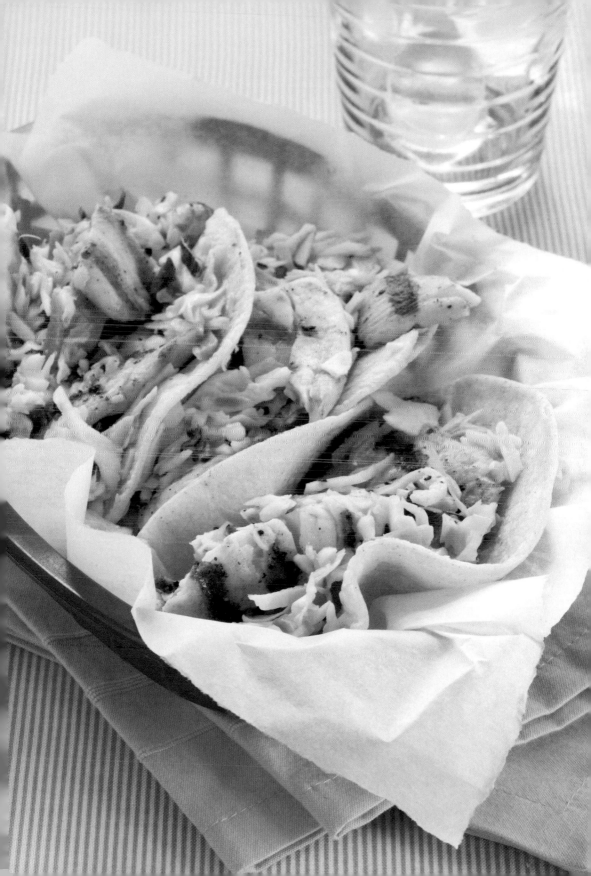

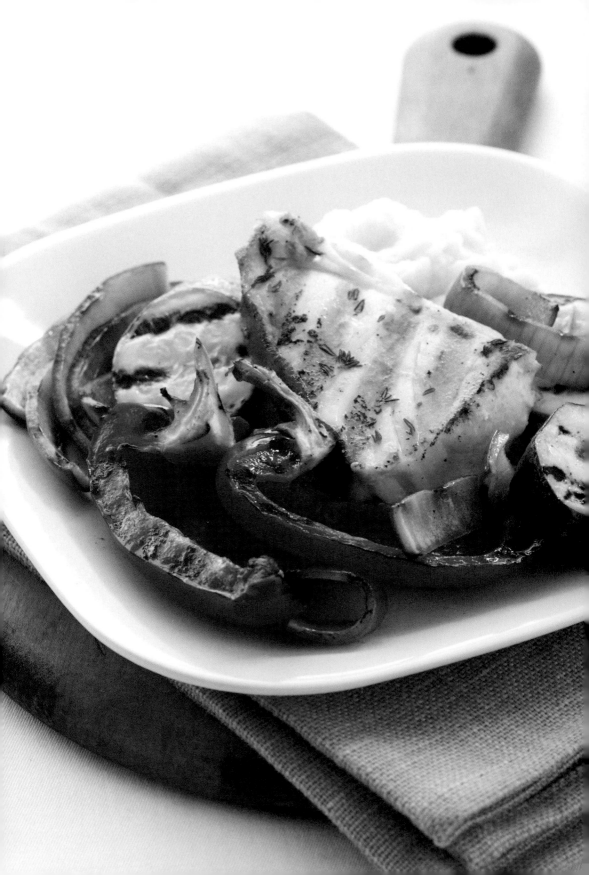

Mediterranean Seafood Grill with Skordalia

This dish includes a slice of sourdough bread in the garlicky potato sauce known as skordalia. This thick and creamy sauce can also be used as a spread on sandwiches or as a dip for veggies and rye crackers.

PREP: 15 minutes
COOK: 40 minutes
TOTAL TIME: 55 minutes
MAKES: 4 servings

Resistant Starch: 1.7g

- 1 **pound russet or Yukon gold potatoes, peeled and diced**
- 8 **garlic cloves, peeled**
- 1 **slice sourdough bread, crust removed, and torn into pieces**
- ¼ **cup plain low-fat Greek yogurt**
- 3 **tablespoons olive oil, divided**
  Zest and juice of 1 lemon
- ½ **teaspoon salt, divided**
- ¼ **teaspoon dried thyme**
- 1 **pound halibut fillets, cut into 4 pieces**
- 2 **red bell peppers, quartered**
- 1 **pound small zucchini, diagonally cut into 1-inch pieces**
- ½ **red onion, sliced**

1. Place potatoes in a large saucepan, add garlic, cover with cold water, and cook over high heat 15 minutes or until potatoes are tender.

2. While the potatoes cook, place the bread in a large bowl. Spoon 2–3 tablespoons cooking liquid from potatoes over bread. Stir with a fork until smooth. Add yogurt, 2 tablespoons olive oil, and lemon zest and juice; stir until a smooth paste forms.

3. Place a large bowl in the sink, and set a colander on top. Drain potatoes and garlic, reserving cooking liquid. Transfer potatoes to bread mixture, and mash until smooth. Add reserved cooking liquid 2 tablespoons at a time until mixture takes on the consistency of loose mashed potatoes. Stir in ¼ teaspoon salt and 2 teaspoons olive oil. Cover and keep warm.

4. Preheat grill pan over medium-high heat. Drizzle fish with ½ teaspoon olive oil, and sprinkle with remaining ¼ teaspoon salt and thyme. Cook 2–3 minutes on each side or until fish flakes easily with a fork. Transfer to a plate; cover and keep warm.

5. Place bell pepper, zucchini, and red onion in a large bowl. Drizzle with remaining ½ teaspoon olive oil; toss to coat. Arrange bell pepper in grill pan, and cook 5 minutes over medium heat. Add zucchini and onion; cook 10 minutes or until vegetables are tender, turning as necessary for even cooking.

6. Serve halibut with grilled vegetables and skordalia.

Serving size: 4 ounces halibut, ¼ of grilled vegetables, and ½ cup skordalia | Calories 390; Fat 14g (sat 2g, mono 8g, poly 2g); Cholesterol 35mg; Protein 31g; Carbohydrate 37g; Sugars 7g; Fiber 5g; RS 1.7g; Sodium 280mg

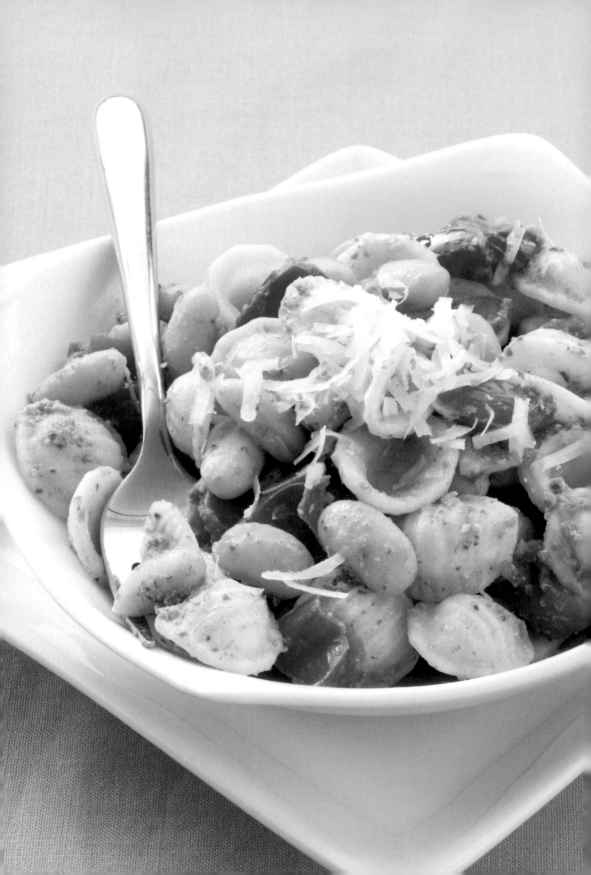

Orecchiette with White Beans & Pesto

You can use any small pasta for this dish. Letting it cool to room temperature before serving will boost the Resistant Starch factor even higher.

PREP: 10 minutes
COOK: 15 minutes
TOTAL TIME: 25 minutes
MAKES: 4 servings

Resistant Starch:
4.4g

1 **cup uncooked orecchiette or seashell pasta**
1 **teaspoon olive oil**
2 **garlic cloves, minced**
1 **(15-ounce) can white kidney beans, rinsed and drained**
3 **plum tomatoes, chopped (about 1½ cups)**
⅓ **cup prepared pesto**
¼ **cup shredded Parmesan cheese**

1. Cook pasta according to package directions, omitting salt and fat.

2. While the pasta cooks, heat olive oil and garlic in a large nonstick skillet over medium-high heat until garlic is fragrant. Add beans and tomato; reduce heat to low, and cook, stirring occasionally, about 5–7 minutes.

3. Drain pasta, and add to bean mixture. Add pesto; toss to combine. Divide evenly among 4 servings dishes. Top each serving with 1 table-spoon Parmesan cheese.

Serving size: 1¼ cups | Calories 420; Fat 11g (sat 2.5g, mono 4g, poly 5g); Cholesterol 5mg; Protein 18g; Carbohydrate 63g; Sugars 5g; Fiber 7g; RS 4.4g; Sodium 360mg

Pan-Seared Scallops with Southwestern Rice Salad

For an extra metabolism boost, feel free to add a kick of hot sauce, cayenne, jalapeños, or chilies to this dish.

PREP: 20 minutes
COOK: 10 minutes
TOTAL TIME: 30 minutes
MAKES: 4 servings

Resistant Starch:
3.7g

- 1 lime
- 2 teaspoons olive oil, divided
- 1 teaspoon chili powder, divided
- ½ teaspoon salt, divided
- 1 (15-ounce) can low-sodium black beans, rinsed and drained
- 1 (11-ounce) can corn, drained
- 1 cup grape tomatoes, halved
- ½ cup chopped scallions
- 2 tablespoons chopped fresh cilantro
- 3 cups cooked brown rice
- 1 pound dry scallops (about 16)

1. Squeeze juice from half the lime into a large bowl; add 1 teaspoon olive oil, ½ teaspoon chili powder, and ¼ teaspoon salt; stir well with a whisk. Add beans, corn, tomato, scallions, and cilantro; toss gently to combine. Stir in cooked rice, and toss until thoroughly combined. Cover loosely, and keep warm.

2. Combine remaining 1 teaspoon olive oil, remaining ½ teaspoon chili powder, and remaining ¼ teaspoon salt in a large bowl. Pat scallops dry with a paper towel, and add to oil mixture, tossing until thoroughly coated. Squeeze 2 teaspoons juice from remaining lime half into a small bowl, and set aside.

3. Heat a large nonstick skillet over medium-high heat. Arrange scallops in pan, flat sides down (make sure they aren't touching or they will steam, not sear properly). Cook 2–3 minutes on each side until lightly browned and opaque in the center. Drizzle scallops with reserved lime juice, and toss gently to coat. Divide rice mixture evenly among 4 serving dishes, and top each serving with 4 scallops. Serve immediately.

Serving size: 4 scallops and 1½ cups rice salad | Calories 419; Fat 5g (sat 1g, mono 2g, poly 1g); Cholesterol 37mg; Protein 30g; Carbohydrate 64g; Sugars 4g; Fiber 9g; RS 3.7g; Sodium 497mg

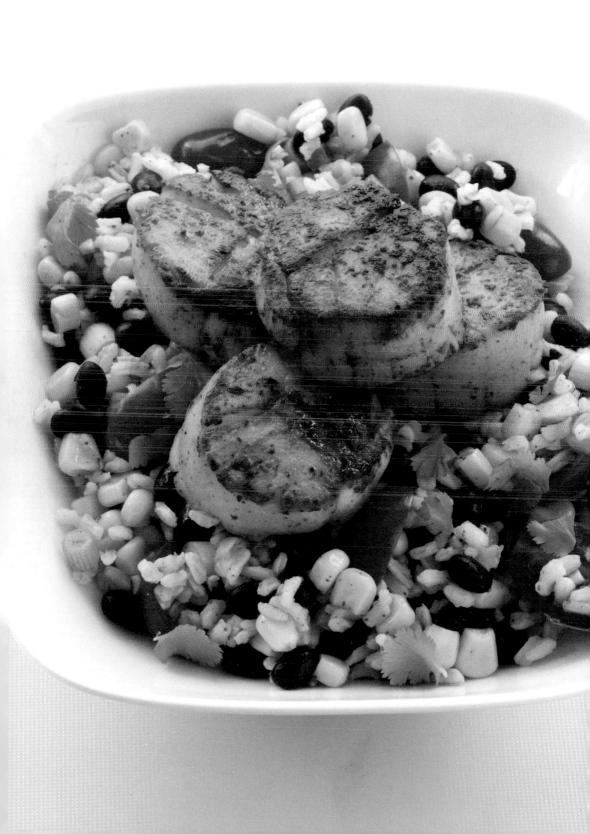

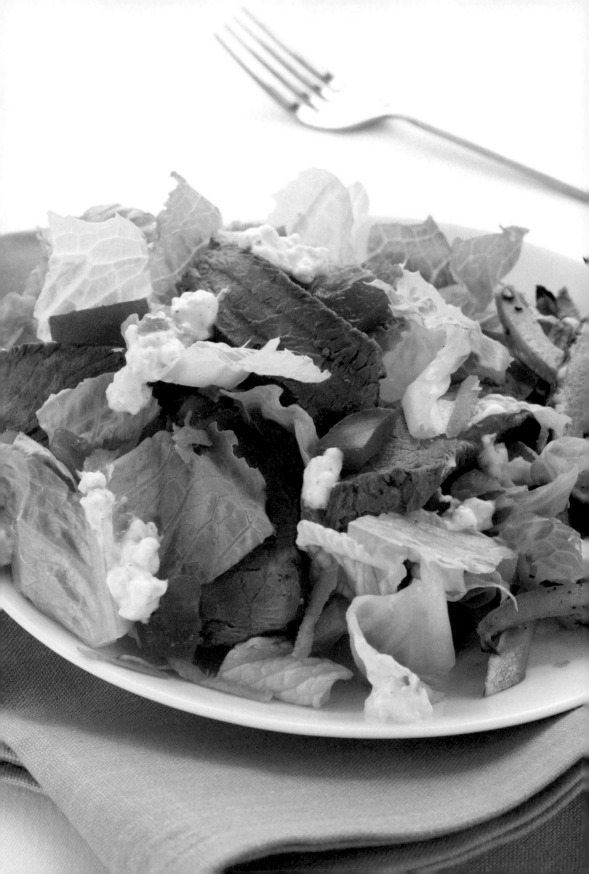

Sirloin Salad with Blue Cheese Dressing & Sweet Potato Fries

Blue cheese? Steak? Fries?! Is this diet food? Yes! By baking the fries, you slash calories without sacrificing flavor. Save time by using frozen sweet potato fries.

PREP: 10 minutes
COOK: 20 minutes
TOTAL TIME: 30 minutes
MAKES: 4 servings

Resistant Starch: 2.5g

- 1½ **pounds sweet potatoes, cut into ¼-inch-thick matchsticks**
- 1 **pound sirloin steak**
   Cooking spray
- ½ **teaspoon salt, divided**
- ½ **teaspoon pepper, divided**
- ½ **cup plain low-fat Greek yogurt**
- 4 **tablespoons crumbled blue cheese**
- 8 **cups chopped Romaine lettuce**
- 2 **tomatoes, diced**
- 2 **carrots, peeled and shredded**

1. Preheat broiler. Coat sweet potato fries and steak with cooking spray. Place on separate baking sheets, and sprinkle with ¼ teaspoon each salt and pepper. Place fries and steak in oven for 20 minutes, turning fries once, halfway through. Steak is done when a meat thermometer inserted into the thickest part registers 160° (medium). Fries should be tender and crisp.

2. Combine yogurt, blue cheese, and remaining ¼ teaspoon each salt and pepper. Toss lettuce, tomato, and carrot together.

3. Cut steak into strips. Arrange the salad evenly on 4 plates and top with steak. Drizzle dressing over salad; serve with sweet potato fries.

Serving size: 3 cups salad, 3 ounces steak, 1 cup fries, and 1 tablespoon ketchup | Calories 391; Fat 9g (sat 4g, mono 3g, poly 0.5g); Cholesterol 56mg; Protein 34g; Carbohydrate 44g; Sugars 12g; Fiber 8g; RS 2.5g; Sodium 393mg

Spanish-Style Shrimp with Yellow Rice

Many Spanish dishes call for super-pricey saffron. To save money, we've substituted turmeric, a spice that lends a similar flavor and color for a fraction of the cost.

PREP: 10 minutes
COOK: 15 minutes
TOTAL TIME: 25 minutes
MAKES: 4 servings

Resistant Starch: 3.8g

    4 garlic cloves, minced
    2 tablespoons olive oil, divided
 1½ teaspoons smoked paprika
    ½ teaspoon salt, divided
    1 pound large shrimp, peeled and deveined
    ½ cup finely chopped onion
    3 cups uncooked quick-cooking brown rice
    ½ teaspoon ground turmeric
 2½ cups cold water
    ½ cup frozen peas
    2 tablespoons dry sherry (optional)
    1 tablespoon fresh chopped parsley

1. Combine garlic, 1 tablespoon olive oil, paprika, and ¼ teaspoon salt in a large bowl; stir with a whisk. Add shrimp, and toss to coat. Set aside.

2. Heat remaining 1 tablespoon oil in a 3-quart saucepan over medium-high heat. Add onion, and cook 2–3 minutes until soft. Add rice, remaining ¼ teaspoon salt, and turmeric. Add 2½ cups cold water; cover and reduce heat to low. Cook 4 minutes; remove from heat. Stir in peas, and let stand, covered, until ready to serve.

3. Heat a large nonstick skillet over medium-high heat. Place shrimp in center of pan. Cook 2–3 minutes on each side or until opaque. Add sherry, if desired, during the last minute of cooking, and toss to coat. Remove from heat. Fluff rice mixture, and place on a serving platter. Arrange shrimp on top of rice mixture, sprinkle with parsley, and serve immediately.

Serving size: ¼ of shrimp and 1 cup rice | Calories 430; Fat 10g (sat 1.5g, mono 5g, poly 2g); Cholesterol 170mg; Protein 31g; Carbohydrate 56g; Sugars 1g; Fiber 5g; RS 3.8g; Sodium 470mg

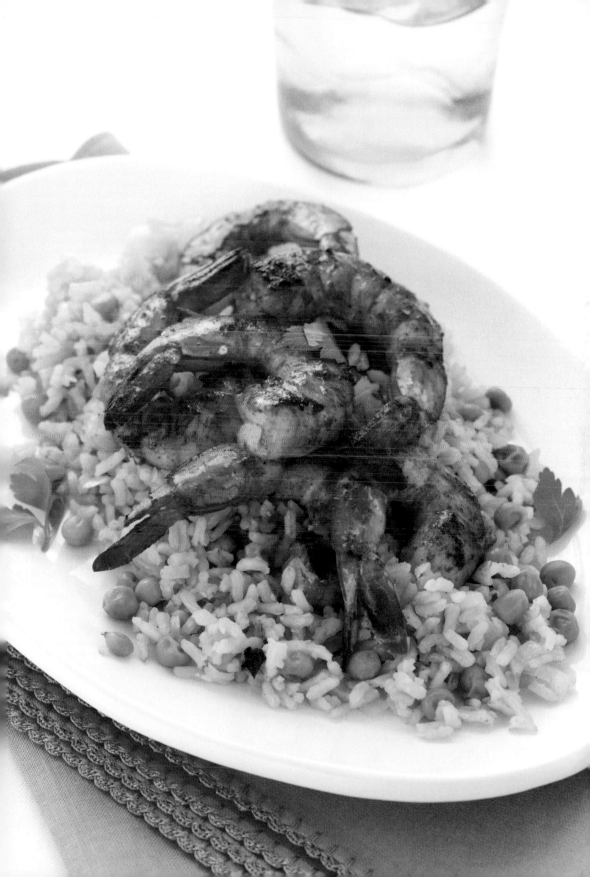

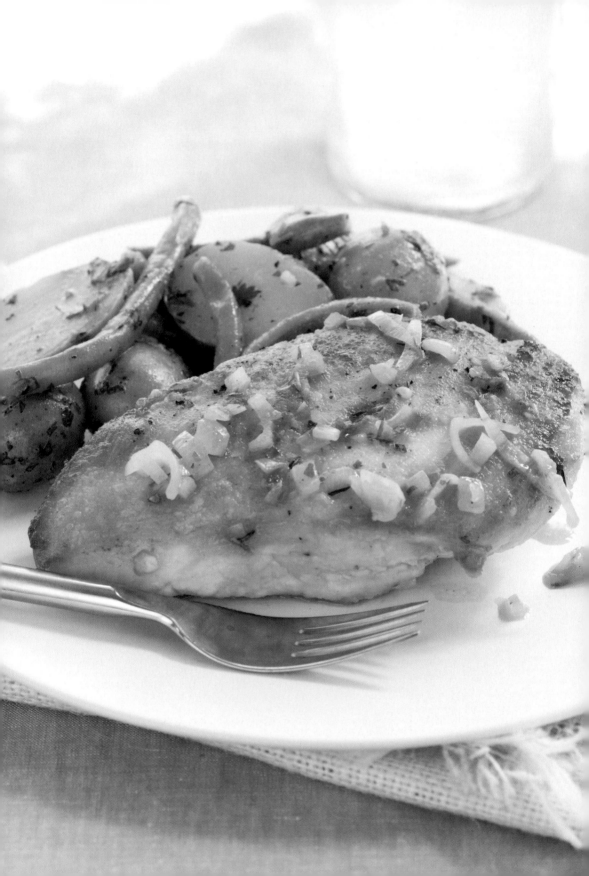

Seared Chicken Breasts with French Potato Salad

Double the amount of Resistant Starch in this dish by allowing the potato salad to cool to room temperature before serving.

PREP: 15 minutes
COOK: 20 minutes
TOTAL TIME: 35 minutes
MAKES: 4 servings

Resistant Starch: **2.3** g

- 1½ pounds baby Yukon gold potatoes
- 1 cup frozen whole green beans
- 2 tablespoons olive oil, divided
- 2 tablespoons chopped fresh parsley
- 1 tablespoon Dijon mustard
- 1 tablespoon cider vinegar
- ½ teaspoon salt, divided
  Freshly ground black pepper
- 4 (5-ounce) skinless, boneless chicken breasts
- 2 tablespoons all-purpose flour
- 1 large shallot, finely chopped (about ½ cup)
- ¼ cup fresh lemon juice
- ½ teaspoon dried tarragon

1. Place potatoes in a large saucepan; cover with water. Bring water to a boil, and cook 15 minutes or until potatoes can be easily pierced with a fork. Add green beans during last minute of cooking; drain and set aside.

2. While potatoes and beans cook, combine 1 tablespoon olive oil, parsley, mustard, vinegar, and ¼ teaspoon salt in a large bowl; stir with a whisk. Season to taste with black pepper. When potatoes are cool enough to handle, slice larger pieces in half, and add to bowl. Toss to coat, and set aside.

3. Cover chicken breasts with parchment paper; pound to an even thickness using a mallet or small, heavy skillet. Sprinkle with remaining ¼ teaspoon salt and season with black pepper.

4. Place flour in a shallow dish; dredge chicken in flour. Heat remaining 1 tablespoon olive oil in a large nonstick skillet over medium-high heat. Add chicken to pan, and cook 6–8 minutes or until chicken begins to brown; turn to brown other side. Add shallots, and cook 5–6 minutes or until a meat thermometer inserted into the thickest part of the chicken breast registers 165°. Add lemon juice and tarragon, and turn chicken until evenly coated.

5. Place chicken breast on each of 4 serving plates; serve with potato salad.

Serving size: 1 chicken breast and 1¼ cups potato salad | Calories 380; Fat 9g (sat 1.5g, mono 5g, poly 1g); Cholesterol 80mg; Protein 37g; Carbohydrate 37g; Sugars 3g; Fiber 5g; RS 2.3g; Sodium 490mg

Roasted Pork Tenderloin with Apricot-Barley Pilaf

Tossing the barley into the pan after the pork is done roasting means that this dish doesn't waste a drop of flavor—and you'll have fewer dishes to wash afterward, too.

PREP: 10 minutes
COOK: 30 minutes
TOTAL TIME: 40 minutes
MAKES: 4 servings

Resistant Starch: **2.9g**

 1 pound pork tenderloin, trimmed of visible fat
 1 teaspoon olive oil
 ¼ teaspoon salt
   Freshly ground black pepper
 2 tablespoons apricot jam
 1 tablespoon less-sodium soy sauce
 ¼ cup pecans, coarsely chopped
 1 celery stalk, finely chopped (about ⅓ cup)
 1 carrot, peeled and diced (about ⅓ cup)
 ¼ cup finely chopped onion
 ¾ cup water
 3 cups quick-cooking barley, cooked
 ½ cup dried apricot halves, chopped
 ¼ cup chopped fresh parsley

1. Preheat oven to 375°.

2. Rub pork with olive oil; sprinkle with salt and pepper, and set aside. Combine jam and soy sauce in a small bowl; set aside.

3. Heat a large ovenproof nonstick skillet over medium-high heat. Add pecans, and cook, tossing frequently, 3–5 minutes or until fragrant.

4. Return pan to heat, and add pork. Cook 5 minutes, turning every minute or two to brown evenly on all sides. Add jam mixture, celery, carrot, and onion to pan; stir until jam melts and vegetables and pork are evenly coated with sauce. Stir in ¾ cup water. Place pan in oven, and bake at 375° for 18–20 minutes or until a meat thermometer inserted into pork registers 160°.

5. Remove pan from oven; transfer pork to plate. Cover loosely with foil, and let stand 5 minutes.

6. Stir barley, apricots, and toasted pecans into vegetable mixture. (Remember the handle of the pan will be very hot!) Stir in parsley. Carefully slice pork into 12 equal pieces. Serve 3 slices pork on top of barley pilaf.

Serving size: 3 pieces pork and 1 cup pilaf | Calories 400; Fat 9g (sat 1.5g, mono 4g, poly 2g); Cholesterol 75mg; Protein 28g; Carbohydrate 54g; Sugars 15g; Fiber 7g; RS 2.9g; Sodium 390mg

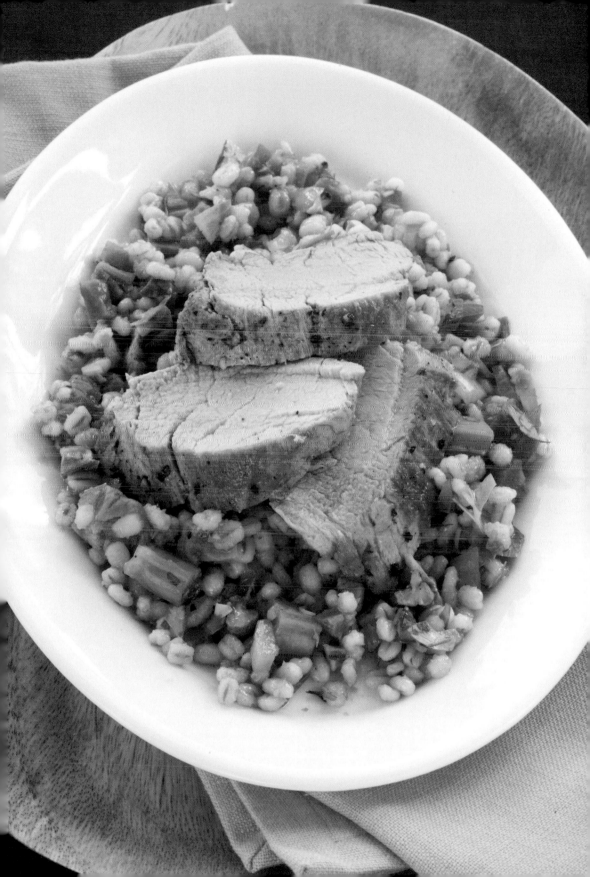

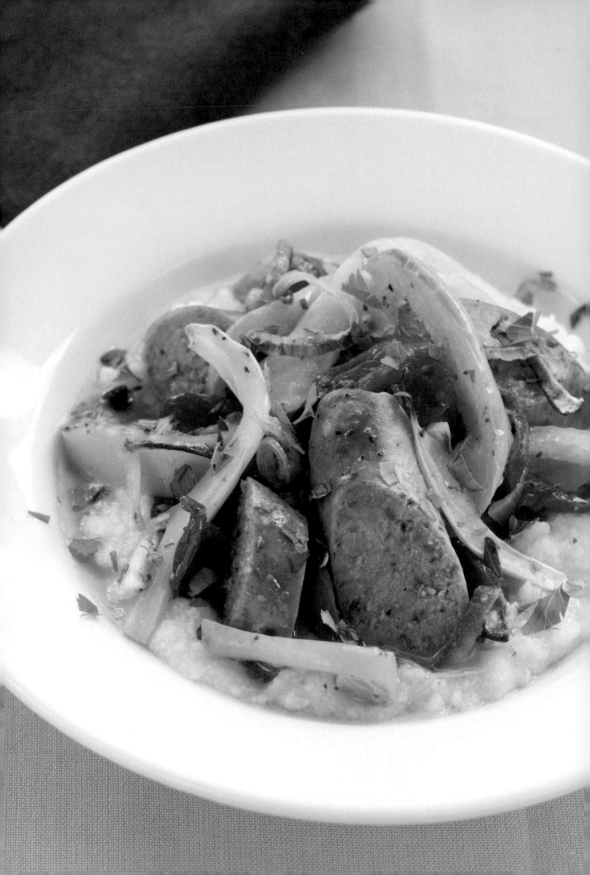

Roasted Vegetables & Italian Sausage with Polenta

We've shrunk the calorie count of this dish by using lean turkey sausage. To save time, use store-bought polenta in a tube.

PREP: 20 minutes
COOK: 1 hour and 15 minutes
TOTAL TIME: 1 hour and 35 minutes
MAKES: 4 servings

Resistant Starch:

2 g

Cooking spray
4 cups water
1 cup polenta
1 small fennel bulb (about ½ pound), stem and fronds removed, sliced thin
1 yellow or orange bell pepper, sliced (about 1 cup)
½ red onion, sliced (about 1 cup)
2 cups grape tomatoes, halved
4 garlic cloves, crushed
1 tablespoon olive oil
½ teaspoon dried oregano
4 (4-ounce) lean Italian turkey sausage links
1 cup water
2 tablespoons fresh chopped parsley (optional)

1. Preheat oven to 425°.

2. Coat a 3-quart baking dish with cooking spray. Combine 4 cups water and polenta, and pour into prepared baking dish. Set aside.

3. Place fennel in a 9- x 13-inch baking dish. Add bell pepper, red onion, tomatoes, and garlic. Drizzle with olive oil, and sprinkle with oregano. Toss to coat. Arrange turkey sausage on top, and add 1 cup water.

4. Bake sausage and vegetables, uncovered, at 425° for 20 minutes. Remove from oven; turn sausages, and toss vegetables. Place half of vegetable mixture on top of sausages before returning baking dish to oven.

5. Reduce temperature to 350°. Stir polenta mixture lightly, and place baking dish in oven. Bake at 350° for 45 minutes. Remove polenta from oven; stir gently with a fork, and return to oven. Bake both dishes an additional 10 minutes or until vegetables are completely soft and a thermometer inserted into the thickest part of a sausage registers 170°. Remove from oven.

6. Stir polenta with a fork; polenta will continue to thicken as it stands. Serve polenta and sausage topped with vegetables and pan sauce. Sprinkle with parsley, if desired.

Serving size: 1 cup polenta, 1 sausage, ½ cup vegetables, and 2 tablespoons pan sauce | Calories 390; Fat 14g (sat 3g, mono 2.5g, poly 0g); Cholesterol 76mg; Protein 25g; Carbohydrate 41g; Sugars 4g; Fiber 5g; RS 2g; Sodium 498mg

Thai Peanut Noodles

Resistant
Starch:
2 _g_

Supplying half your daily requirement for fiber, lots of appetite-suppressing protein, and some Resistant Starch and MUFAs, this quick-and-simple Asian-themed dish is just as slimming as it is satisfying.

PREP: 15 minutes
COOK: 15 minutes
TOTAL TIME: 30 minutes
MAKES: 4 servings

8 **ounces uncooked whole-wheat linguine**
2 **cups broccoli florets**
1 **cup shelled frozen edamame**
½ **cup peanut satay sauce (such as Thai Kitchen)**
2 **cups bean sprouts**
1 **large carrot, peeled and shredded**
½ **red bell pepper, cut into thin slices**
¼ **cup lightly salted, dry-roasted peanuts, chopped**
Fresh lime wedges

1. Cook pasta according to package directions, omitting salt and fat. During the last minute of cooking, add broccoli and edamame. Drain well, and transfer to a large bowl.

2. Add satay sauce to pasta mixture, and toss to coat. Add bean sprouts, carrot, and bell pepper; toss until thoroughly combined. Divide pasta mixture evenly among 4 serving plates; top each serving with 1 tablespoon chopped peanuts. Serve with lime wedges.

Serving size: 2½ cups | Calories 410; Fat 13g (sat 2g, mono 2g, poly 2g); Cholesterol 0mg; Protein 21g; Carbohydrate 61g; Sugars 8g; Fiber 14g; RS 2g; Sodium 610mg

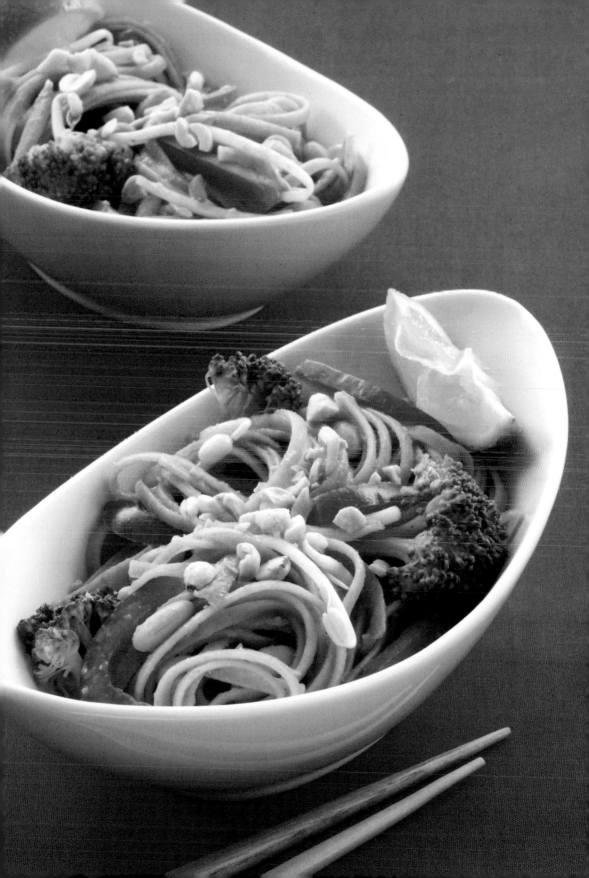

Baked Two-Cheese Penne with Roasted Red Pepper Sauce

You'll love this twist on traditional macaroni and cheese, and so will your kids. Cheese adds fat-burning CLA.

PREP: 10 minutes
COOK: 35 minutes
TOTAL TIME: 45 minutes
MAKES: 4 servings

Resistant Starch:

2g

Cooking spray
1 cup uncooked whole-wheat penne
2 tablespoons olive oil
2 tablespoons all-purpose flour
½ teaspoon salt
¼ teaspoon freshly ground black pepper
1½ cups 1% low-fat milk
1 ounce smoked Gouda, shredded (about ¼ cup)
2 ounces fontina cheese, shredded (about ½ cup)
¼ cup panko (Japanese breadcrumbs)
½ cup roasted red bell pepper
1 tablespoon plain low-fat Greek yogurt

1. Heat oven to 350°. Coat an 8-inch square baking dish with cooking spray; set aside.

2. Bring a large pot of water to a boil over high heat; add pasta, and cook 7 minutes or until al dente. Drain and set aside.

3. Reduce heat to medium, and add olive oil to pan. Add flour, salt, and pepper; cook 1–2 minutes until flour begin to brown. Stir in milk, ½ cup at a time, whisking well to ensure a smooth sauce. Stir in cheeses; whisk until completely melted. Stir in cooked pasta. Transfer mixture to prepared baking dish.

4. Top pasta mixture with panko; bake at 350° for 20 minutes or until top begins to brown and cheese is bubbly.

5. While pasta mixture bakes, place roasted bell pepper and yogurt in a blender or food processor; process until smooth. Cut baked pasta evenly into 4 pieces, and place on 4 serving dishes; drizzle each serving with roasted red pepper sauce.

Serving size: ¼ of penne and 2 tablespoons sauce | Calories 433; Fat 16g (sat 6g, mono 7g, poly 1g); Cholesterol 29mg; Protein 17g; Carbohydrate 56g; Sugars 8g; Fiber 5g; RS 2g; Sodium 528mg

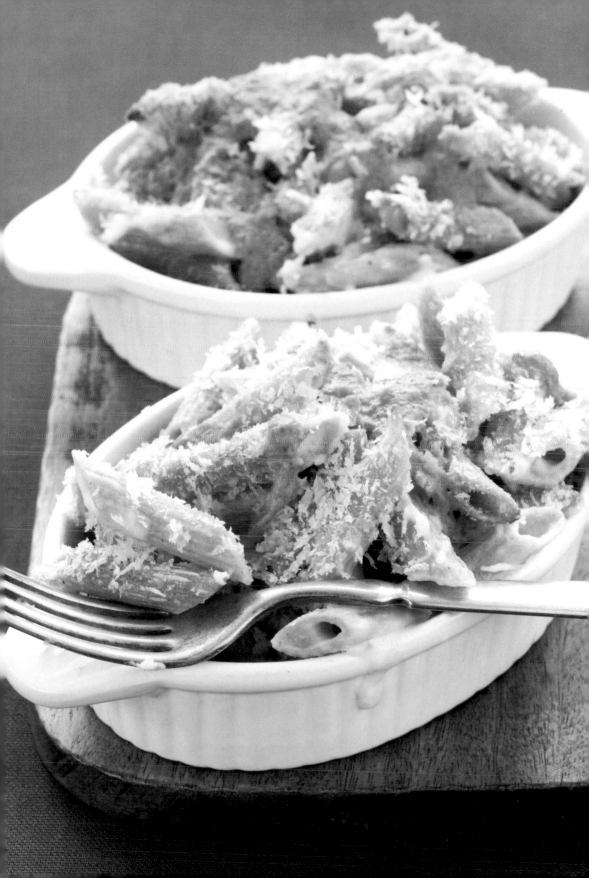

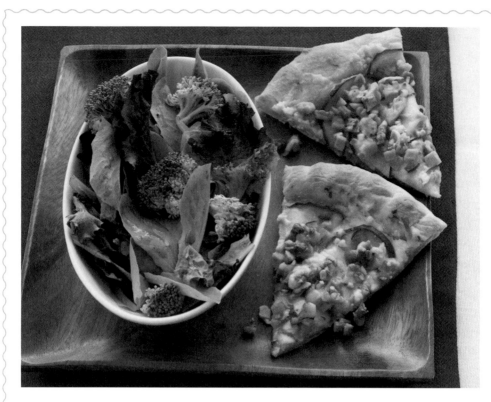

Bacon, Pear & Gorgonzola Pizza

If you don't want to make your own pizza dough, go ahead and use prepared—or even a whole-wheat pita bread.

PREP: 15 minutes
COOK: 20 minutes
TOTAL TIME: 35 minutes
MAKES: 4 servings

- 8 **ounces store-bought pizza dough (or make your own with our recipe on the next page)**
- ⅓ **cup part-skim ricotta cheese**
- 1 **tablespoon honey**
- ½ **cup shredded part-skim mozzarella cheese, divided**
- 1 **pear, halved, cored, and thinly sliced**
- 2 **ounces Canadian bacon, finely chopped**
- ¼ **cup chopped walnuts**
- 2 **tablespoons crumbled gorgonzola or other blue cheese**
- 6 **cups mixed greens, divided**
- 2 **cups broccoli florets, divided**
- 6 **tablespoons low-fat balsamic vinaigrette, divided**

1. Preheat oven to 400°.

2. With a floured rolling pin, roll dough into a 12-inch circle; transfer to a 12-inch pizza stone or round baking pan. Bake at 400° for 5–7 minutes or until crust begins to puff.

3. While crust bakes, stir together ricotta cheese and honey. Remove crust from oven, and flip so bottom is now on top. Spread ricotta mixture evenly over crust. Top with ¼ cup mozzarella, pear, Canadian bacon, and walnuts. Top with remaining ¼ cup mozzarella and gorgonzola.

4. Return pizza to oven; bake an additional 15 minutes until cheese is melted and bubbly. Allow pizza to set before slicing into 8 pieces.

5. While pizza bakes, assemble side salads, using 1½ cups greens, ½ cup broccoli, and 1½ tablespoons dressing per serving.

Serving size: 2 slices pizza and 2 cups salad | Calories 360; Fat 13g (sat 4.5g, mono 3g, poly 4g); Cholesterol 24mg; Protein 17g; Carbohydrate 46g; Sugars 12g; Fiber 7g; RS 1.6g; Sodium 504mg

Pizza Dough
PREP: 10 minutes with 1 hour rising time
TOTAL TIME: 1 hour 10 minutes
MAKES: 1½ pounds dough (enough for 3 thin 12-inch pizzas; 12 servings)

> 1 **cup warm water (about 110°)**
> 2 **teaspoons (about 1 package) active dry yeast**
> 1 **teaspoon sugar**
> 2 **cups all-purpose flour**
> 1 **cup whole-wheat or white flour**
> ½ **teaspoon salt**
> 1 **tablespoon olive oil, divided**

1. Combine warm water, yeast, and sugar in a small bowl; let stand about 10 minutes or until yeast begins to foam.

2. Combine flours and salt in bowl of a stand mixer fitted with a dough hook. Add yeast mixture and 2 teaspoons olive oil. Mix on low speed 2–3 minutes or until dough has formed a ball and no longer feels sticky. Coat dough and insides of bowl with remaining 1 teaspoon olive oil. Cover with a towel, and let rise in a warm place (85°), free from drafts, about 1 hour or until doubled in size.

3. Refrigerate unused dough for up to 3 days in a zip-top plastic bag.

CarbLovers Immersion
Snack Recipes

Coconut-Date Truffles

For best results, use Medjool dates for this recipe; they are extra plump and moist. You can store leftover truffles covered in the fridge for up to 10 days.

Resistant Starch:
0.2 g

PREP: 10 minutes
TOTAL TIME: 10 minutes
MAKES: 4 servings

- 8 dates, pitted and chopped
- 8 tablespoons puffed-wheat cereal
- 2 tablespoons shredded coconut

1. Place dates in a large bowl. Mash with fingers until dates form a ball.

2. Add cereal; knead into dates.

3. Form into 8 balls; roll each in coconut to coat.

Serving size: 2 truffles | Calories 160; Fat 2g (sat 1.5g, mono 0g, poly 0g); Cholesterol 0mg; Protein 1g; Carbohydrate 38g; Sugars 32g; Fiber 4g; RS 0.2g; Sodium 0mg

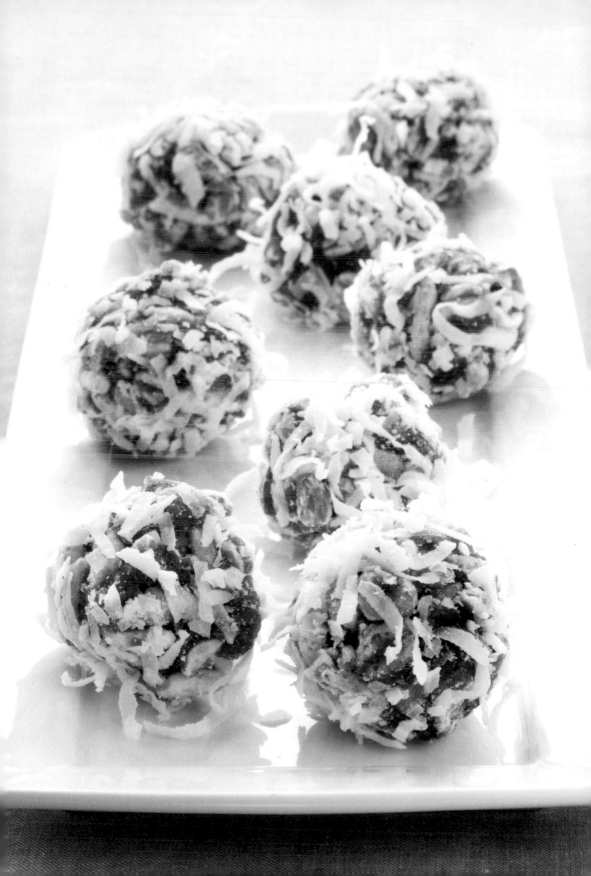

Pea & Walnut Hummus

Resistant Starch: 1.4 g

Usually, hummus is made from chickpeas, but this version uses green peas, which are packed with Resistant Starch and fiber.

PREP: 10 minutes
TOTAL TIME: 10 minutes
MAKES: 4 servings

- 1 **cup frozen peas, thawed**
- 4 **tablespoons chopped walnuts**
- 2 **tablespoons fresh lemon juice**
- 1 **garlic clove, minced**
- ½ **teaspoon salt**
- ½ **teaspoon pepper**
- 8 **rye crispbread crackers**

1. Combine first 6 ingredients (through pepper) in a blender or food processor; process until smooth.

2. Serve with crackers.

Serving size: 2 tablespoons hummus and 2 crackers | Calories 150; Fat 5g (sat 0g, mono 0.5g, poly 3.5g); Cholesterol 0mg; Protein 5g; Carbohydrate 23g; Sugars 1g; Fiber 5g; RS 1.4g; Sodium 340mg

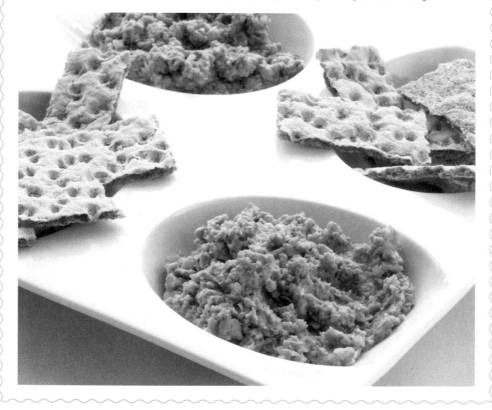

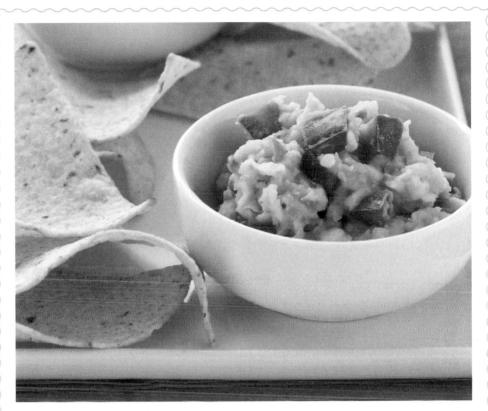

White Bean Salsa & Chips

This easy snack gets you almost a third of your way to your Resistant Starch goal for the day. It serves four, so make up a batch, and store leftovers, covered, in the fridge.

PREP: 10 minutes
TOTAL TIME: 10 minutes
MAKES: 4 servings

- 1 **(15.5-ounce) can white kidney beans, rinsed and drained**
- 2 **tablespoons fresh lime juice**
- ¼ **teaspoon salt**
- 1 **plum tomato, diced**
- 2 **scallions, finely diced**
- 20 **corn chips**

1. Combine beans, juice, and salt in a bowl. Mash with a potato masher until semismooth.

2. Add tomato and scallions; stir to blend. Serve with chips.

Serving size: ¼ cup salsa and 5 chips | Calories 170; Fat 4g (sat 0.5g, mono 0, poly 0g); Cholesterol 0mg; Protein 7g; Carbohydrate 20g; Sugars 1g; Fiber 5g; RS 3g; Sodium 230mg

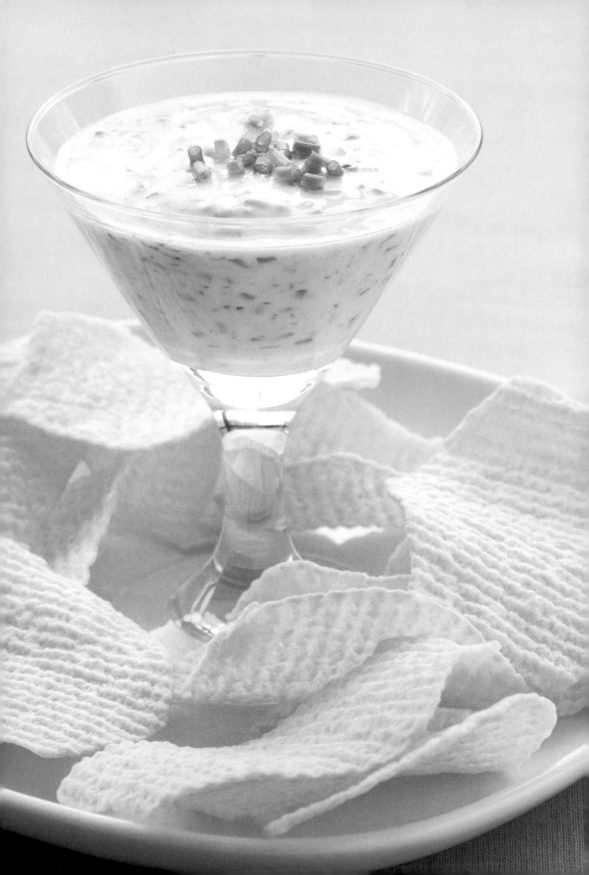

Garlic & Herb Yogurt Dip

If you can't find the thicker, creamier Greek yogurt, substitute plain low-fat yogurt instead. Store leftover dip, covered, in the fridge for up to three days.

PREP: 5 minutes
TOTAL TIME: 5 minutes
MAKES: 4 serving

Resistant Starch: 1 g

- ¾ cup plain low-fat Greek yogurt
- 1 garlic clove, minced
- 2 tablespoons chopped chives
- ¼ teaspoon salt
- ¼ teaspoon pepper
- ¼ teaspoon dried dill
- 1 tablespoon lemon juice
- 4 ounces baked potato chips

1. Combine first 7 ingredients (through lemon juice) in a small bowl. Serve with chips.

Serving size: 3 tablespoons dip and 1 ounce chips (about 12 chips) | Calories 160; Fat 6g (sat 1.5g, mono 3g, poly 1g); Cholesterol 5mg; Protein 5g; Carbohydrate 23g; Sugars 3g; Fiber 1g; RS 1g; Sodium 420mg

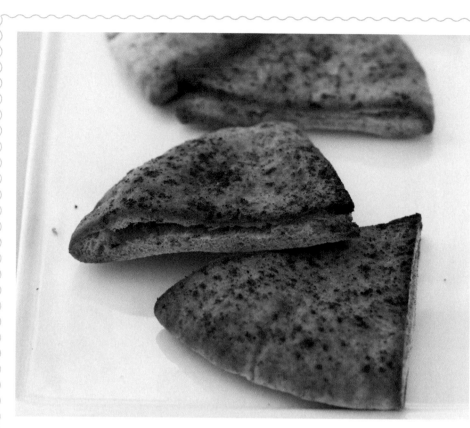

Chili-Spiked Pita Chips

These spicy chips will jump-start your metabolism, satisfy your craving for something crunchy, and supply you with a little Resistant Starch, too.

PREP: 5 minutes
COOK: 5 minutes
TOTAL TIME: 10 minutes
MAKES: 1 serving

> 1 **whole-grain pita**
> **Cooking spray**
> ¼ **teaspoon chili powder**

1. Coat pita with cooking spray; sprinkle with chili powder. Cut pita into 6 triangles.

2. Toast triangles on baking sheet 5 minutes in toaster oven or broiler, turning once, until golden and crunchy.

Serving size: 6 pita chips | Calories 160; Fat 3.5g (sat 0g, mono 0g, poly 1g); Cholesterol 0mg; Protein 6g; Carbohydrate 28g; Sugars 2g; Fiber 4g; RS 1g; Sodium 330mg

Sunflower-Lentil Spread

Lentils are a powerhouse provider of Resistant Starch. In this recipe, they help you get nearly a third of your way to your daily 10-gram goal.

PREP: 10 minutes
TOTAL TIME: 10 minutes
MAKES: 4 servings

Resistant Starch: 3.1g

- 1 (15-ounce) can lentils, rinsed and drained
- 1 tablespoon lemon juice
- ¼ teaspoon salt
- ¼ teaspoon pepper
- 2 tablespoons sunflower seeds
- 1 celery stalk, finely diced
- 1 scallion, finely diced
- 2 tablespoons chopped fresh parsley
- 2 pitas, halved

1. Combine lentils, juice, salt, and pepper in a blender; process until smooth. Stir in sunflower seeds, celery, scallion, and parsley.

2. Microwave pita halves on HIGH 1 minute. Serve with spread.

Serving size: ¼ cup spread and ½ pita | Calories 180; Fat 3g (sat 0g, mono 1g, poly 1.5g); Cholesterol 0mg; Protein 10g; Carbohydrate 29g; Sugars 3g; Fiber 10g; RS 3.1g; Sodium 430mg

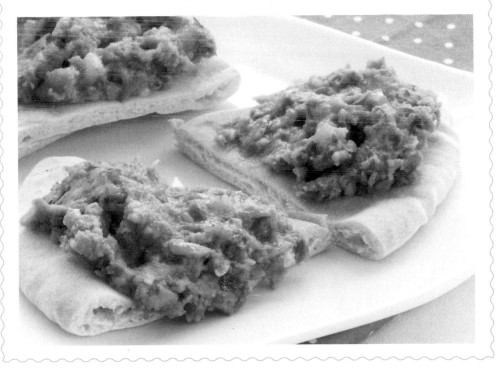

Creamy Sweet Potato Dip

The chipotle chili powder in this sweet and spicy snack will rev your metabolism, while the sweet potato fills you up with Resistant Starch. Speed prep time by using the sweet potato you batch-cooked earlier in the week.

PREP: 5 minutes
BAKE: 10 minutes
TOTAL TIME: 15 minutes
MAKES: 1 serving

Resistant Starch:

2.1 g

- ½ **whole-wheat pita, split and cut into 8 pieces**
- ⅓ **cup roasted mashed sweet potato**
- 1 **tablespoon plain low-fat Greek yogurt**
- ¼ **teaspoon honey**
- ⅛ **teaspoon dried chipotle chile powder**
- ⅛ **teaspoon salt**

1. Preheat oven to 350°. Arrange pita pieces on a baking sheet; bake at 350° for 10 minutes until crisp.

2. While pita bakes, combine sweet potato, yogurt, honey, chile powder, and salt in a small bowl; stir with a fork until smooth. Serve with warm pita chips.

Serving size: ⅓ cup dip and 8 chips | Calories 170; Fat 1g (sat 0g, mono 0g, poly 0.5g); Cholesterol 0mg; Protein 6g; Carbohydrate 35g; Sugars 9g; Fiber 5g; RS 2.1g; Sodium 490mg

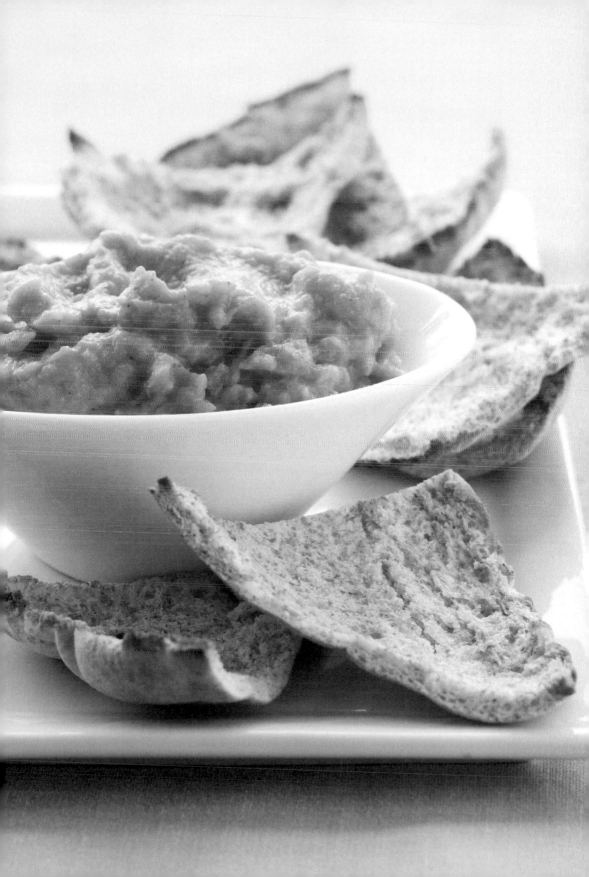

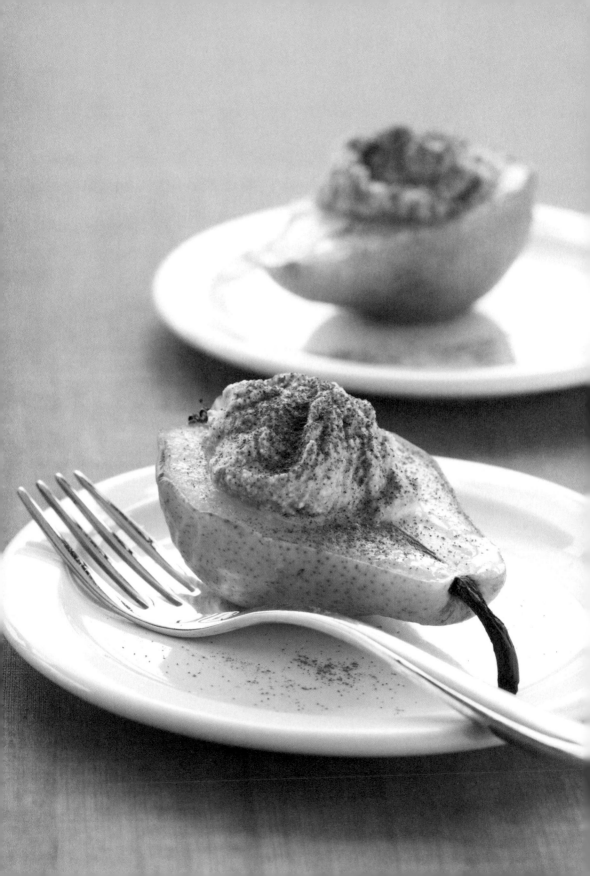

Warm Pear with Cinnamon Ricotta

This snack is rich in both fiber and CLA. The cinnamon is rich in antioxidants and may help control blood sugar, too.

PREP: 5 minutes
COOK: 10 minutes
TOTAL TIME: 15 minutes
MAKES: 1 serving

1 **small pear, halved and cored**
¼ **cup part-skim ricotta cheese**
¼ **teaspoon cinnamon**

1. Preheat broiler or toaster oven. Place pear on a baking sheet; broil 10–12 minutes until tender.

2. Combine ricotta and cinnamon in a small bowl. Top warm pear with ricotta mixture.

Serving size: 1 pear and ¼ cup topping | Calories 170; Fat 5g (sat 3g, mono 1.5g, poly 0g); Cholesterol 20mg; Protein 8g; Carbohydrate 27g; Sugars 15g; Fiber 5g; RS 0g; Sodium 80mg

Cheddar & Apple Melt

In this recipe, sliced apple adds crunch and fiber to a traditional cheese quesadilla.

PREP: 5 minutes
COOK: 5 minutes
TOTAL TIME: 10 minutes
MAKES: 1 serving

Resistant
Starch:
0.8g

- 1 **small apple, thinly sliced**
- 1 **(6-inch) corn tortilla**
- 1 **tablespoon shredded Cheddar cheese**

1. Place apple slices on tortilla. Sprinkle with cheese.

2. Microwave at HIGH 30 seconds until cheese is bubbly. Cut into quarters.

Serving size: 1 melt | Calories 160; Fat 3.5g (sat 1.5g, mono 1g, poly 0.5g); Cholesterol 5mg; Protein 4g; Carbohydrate 31g; Sugars 16g; Fiber 5g; RS 0.8g; Sodium 55mg

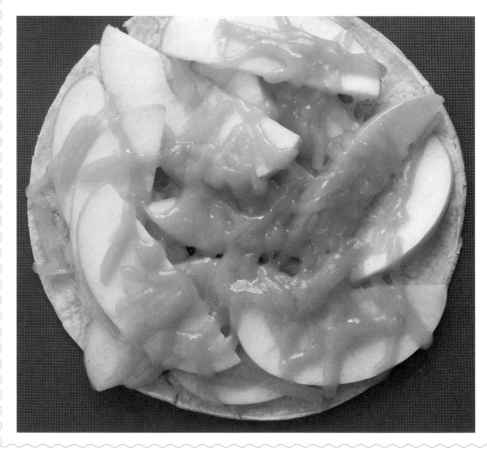

SUPER SIMPLE
CARBLOVERS SNACKS

Easy-to-make snacks are key to *CarbLovers* plan. The 8 snacks listed below can be assembled in about 3 minutes and pack about 150 calories each. They keep your energy up between meals and prevent you from overeating all day.

1. Antipasto Platter: On a serving plate, arrange 12 canned black olives, drained; ½ cup bottled marinated artichoke hearts, drained; and ½ of a bottled roasted red bell pepper, sliced.

2. Pistachio & Dried Cherry Crostini: Combine 2 tablespoons low-fat cottage cheese with 1 teaspoon honey, 2 teaspoons chopped pistachios, and 2 teaspoons chopped dried cherries; serve atop 2 rye crispbread crackers.

3. Brie & Apple Slices: Enjoy 1 small sliced apple with 1 ounce Brie.

4. Fig & Flax Yogurt: Mix ½ cup plain low-fat Greek yogurt with 1 teaspoon honey, 3 chopped dried figs, and 1 teaspoon ground flaxseed.

5. Greek Yogurt with Orange Marmalade & Walnuts: Combine ½ cup plain low-fat Greek yogurt with 2 teaspoons 100-percent fruit orange marmalade and 1 tablespoon chopped walnuts.

6. Honey-Curried Yogurt Dip with Carrots & Broccoli: Combine ½ cup plain low-fat Greek yogurt with 1 teaspoon honey, ¼ teaspoon curry powder, and ⅛ teaspoon salt; serve with ½ cup each baby carrots and broccoli florets.

7. Hummus with Feta & Dill: Top 4 tablespoons store-bought hummus with 1 tablespoon Feta cheese and ⅛ teaspoon dried dill; serve with 1 cup sliced cucumber.

8. Salmon & Cream Cheese Bites: Spread 2 teaspoons low-fat cream cheese on 1 slice toasted pumpernickel bread; top with ½ ounce smoked salmon and 2 teaspoons chopped chives.

CarbLovers Immersion Dessert Recipes

Banana Ice Cream

Resistant Starch:
4 g

Homemade ice cream is easier than you ever imagined! More important, this version is low in sugar and calories and high in omega-3s, fiber, and Resistant Starch.

PREP: 5 minutes
TOTAL TIME: 5 minutes
MAKES: 1 serving

1 small banana, peeled, sliced, and frozen
3 tablespoons 1% low-fat milk
1 tablespoon chopped walnuts

1. Place frozen banana pieces and milk in a blender or food processor; process until thick. Top with walnuts.

Serving size: ½ cup | Calories 160; Fat 6g (sat 1g, mono 1g, poly 3.5g); Cholesterol 0mg; Protein 4g; Carbohydrate 26g; Sugars 15g; Fiber 3g; RS 4g; Sodium 20mg

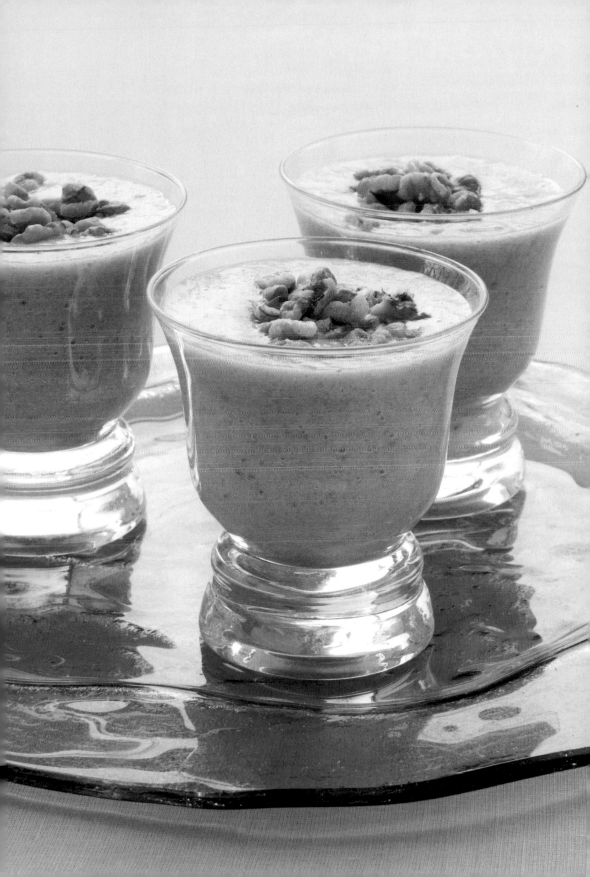

Chocolate-Dipped Banana Bites

Chocolate is a rich source of metabolism-boosting MUFAs, and bananas are the richest source of Resistant Starch there is, making this dessert a weight-loss winner.

PREP: 5 minutes
COOK: 5 minutes
TOTAL TIME: 10 minutes
MAKES: 1 serving

Resistant Starch:

4 g

2 tablespoons semisweet chocolate chips
1 small banana, peeled and cut into 1-inch chunks

1. Place chocolate chips in a small microwave-safe bowl. Microwave on HIGH 1 minute or until chocolate melts. Dip banana pieces halfway in melted chocolate. Serve immediately.

Serving size: 1 banana | Calories 190; Fat 7g (sat 4g, mono 2g, poly 0.5g); Cholesterol 0mg; Protein 2g; Carbohydrate 36g; Sugars 24g; Fiber 4g; RS 4g; Sodium 0mg

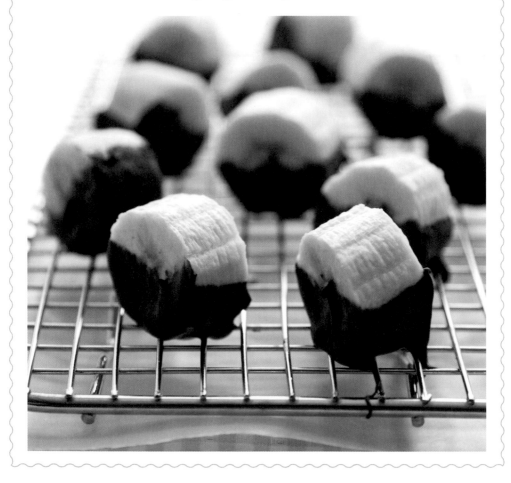

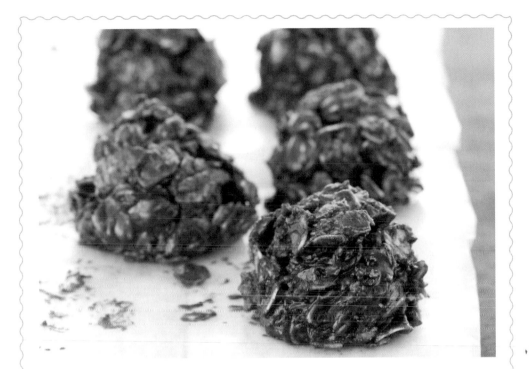

Dark Chocolate & Oat Clusters

What's not to love about chocolate and peanut butter, especially when both are high in MUFAs? As a bonus, the oats provide Resistant Starch.

PREP: 5 minutes
COOK: 3 minutes
STAND: 10 minutes
TOTAL TIME: 18 minutes
MAKES: 4 servings

Resistant Starch:
1.7g

2 **tablespoons peanut butter**
2 **tablespoons 1% low-fat milk**
¼ **cup semisweet chocolate chips**
¾ **cup old-fashioned rolled oats**

1. Heat peanut butter, milk, and chocolate chips in a saucepan over low heat 3 minutes or until chips melt.

2. Stir in oats. Remove from heat.

3. With a spoon, small ice-cream scoop, or melon baller, drop 8 ball-shaped portions on a wax paper–lined baking sheet. Let set in fridge for 10 minutes before serving.

Serving size: 2 clusters | Calories 160; Fat 8g (sat 3g, mono 3.5g, poly 1.5g); Cholesterol 0mg; Protein 5g; Carbohydrate 19g; Sugars 7g; Fiber 3g; RS 1.7g; Sodium 40mg

Chocolate-Orange Spoonbread

Resistant Starch–rich cornmeal gives this dish a deliciously creamy texture.

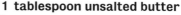

PREP: 5 minutes
COOK: 45 minutes
TOTAL TIME: 50 minutes
MAKES: 6 servings

Resistant Starch:

1 g

- 1 tablespoon unsalted butter
- ⅓ cup sugar
- ¾ cup fine cornmeal
- 2½ cups cold water
- 3 ounces 70-percent dark chocolate, chopped
- Zest of 1 orange (about 1 teaspoon)
- Orange slices for garnish, optional

1. Preheat oven to 350°.

2. Spread butter along bottom and sides of a 3-quart baking dish. Add sugar, cornmeal, and 2½ cups cold water; stir well with a whisk. Bake at 350° for 30 minutes. Remove from oven, and stir mixture carefully with a fork or whisk until smooth; bake an additional 15 minutes.

3. Remove from oven, and stir until smooth. Add chocolate; stir until chocolate melts completely. Garnish with zest, and serve warm or at room temperature with a slice of orange, if desired.

Serving size: ⅓ cup | Calories 200; Fat 8g (sat 5g, mono 2g, poly 0g); Cholesterol 5mg; Protein 2g; Carbohydrate 29g; Sugars 14g; Fiber 4g; RS 1 g; Sodium 12mg

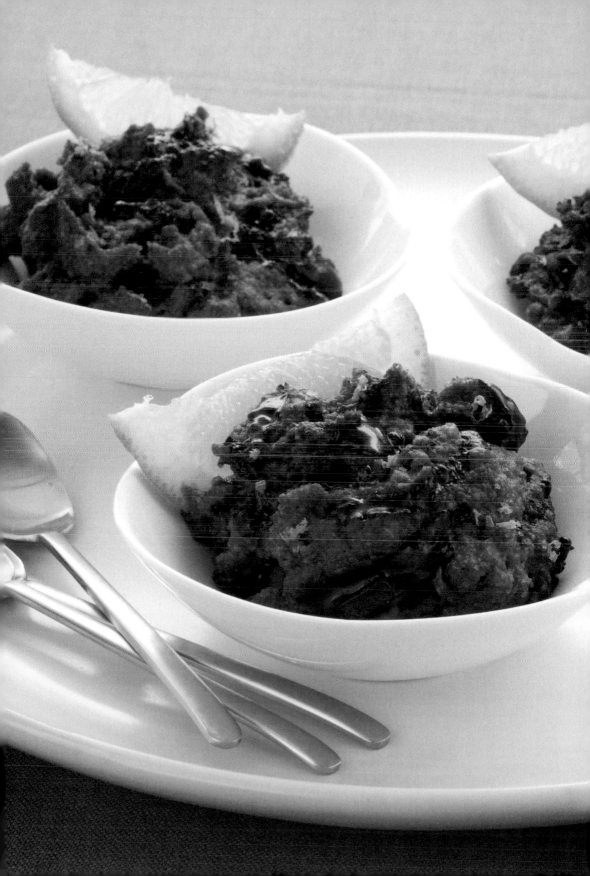

Quick Mango-Coconut Sorbet

It takes almost no time to make this easy sorbet— and it's rich in both fiber and CLA.

PREP: 5 minutes
TOTAL TIME: 5 minutes
MAKES: 1 serving

¾ **cup frozen mango chunks**
3 **tablespoons 1% low-fat milk**
1 **teaspoon honey**
2 **teaspoons shredded coconut, toasted**

1. Place mango, milk, and honey in a blender or food processor; process until thick. Top with coconut.

Serving size: ½ cup | Calories 160; Fat 3g (sat 2.5g, mono 0g, poly 0g); Cholesterol 0mg; Protein 3g; Carbohydrate 33g; Sugars 29g; Fiber 3g; RS 0g; Sodium 20mg

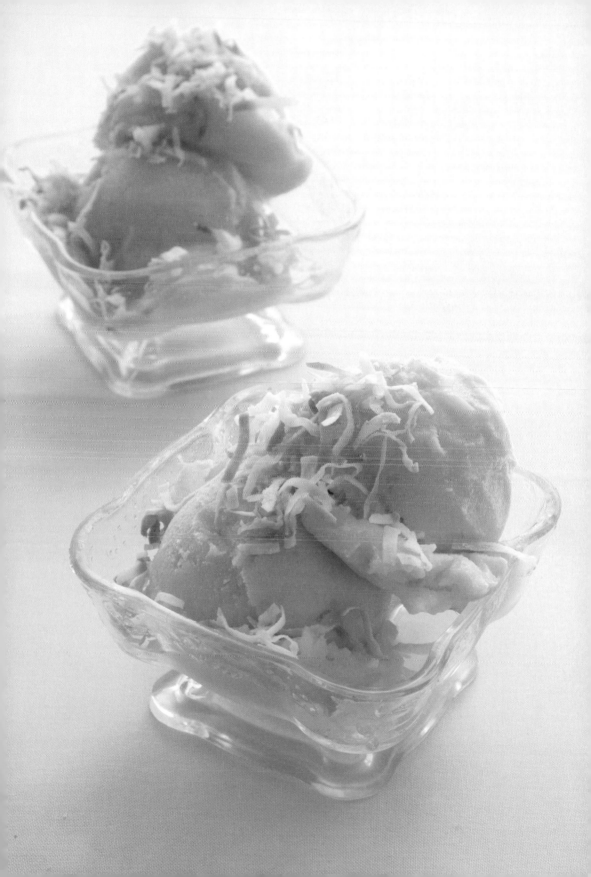

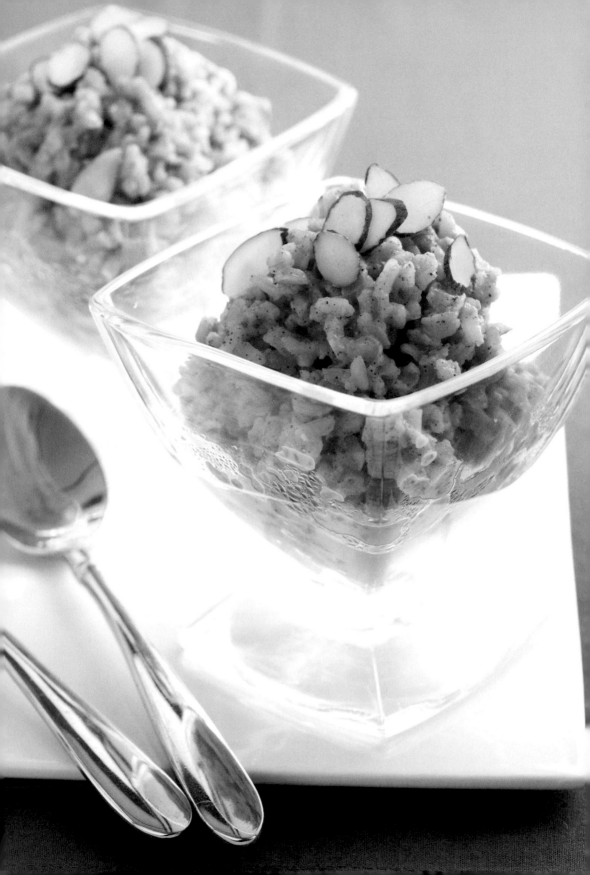

Maple Brown Rice Pudding

This recipe uses Resistant Starch–rich brown rice instead of the usual white. To save time, use a fast-cooking brown rice (such as Uncle Ben's Fast & Natural Instant Whole Grain Brown Rice). The almonds pack metabolism-boosting MUFAs, too, and the cinnamon may help steady blood sugar.

PREP: 5 minutes
COOK: 6 minutes
TOTAL TIME: 11 minutes
MAKES: 4 servings

Resistant Starch:
1.3g

- 1½ **cups cooked brown rice**
- ½ **cup 1% low-fat milk**
- 3 **tablespoons maple syrup**
- ½ **teaspoon ground cinnamon**
- 4 **tablespoons sliced almonds**

1. Combine the rice, milk, maple syrup, and cinnamon in a microwave-safe bowl.

2. Microwave at HIGH 6–8 minutes, stirring occasionally, until most of milk is absorbed. Stir and top with almonds.

Serving size: ½ **cup** | Calories 170; Fat 4g (sat 0.5g, mono 2g, poly 1g); Cholesterol 0mg; Protein 4g; Carbohydrate 30g; Sugars 11g; Fiber 2g; RS 1.3g; Sodium 15mg

Merlot Strawberries with Whipped Cream

Who says wine is just for drinking? You can make an amazing dessert sauce with wine in minutes. Don't worry about getting tipsy: Boiling the sauce removes about 85 percent of the alcohol.

PREP: 5 minutes
COOK: 5 minutes
TOTAL TIME: 10 minutes
MAKES: 4 servings

½ **cup merlot**
2 **tablespoons fresh lemon juice**
2 **tablespoons honey**
¼ **teaspoon vanilla extract**
3 **cups sliced strawberries**
1 **cup whipped cream**

1. Bring merlot, juice, and honey to a boil in a saucepan over high heat. Remove from heat; stir in vanilla.

2. Drizzle sauce over sliced berries. Top with whipped cream.

Serving size: ¾ cup berries, ¼ cup whipped cream, and 2 tablespoons wine sauce | Calories 140; Fat 3.5g (sat 2g, mono 1g, poly 0.5g); Cholesterol 10mg; Protein 1g; Carbohydrate 22g; Sugars 16g; Fiber 3g; RS 0g; Sodium 20mg

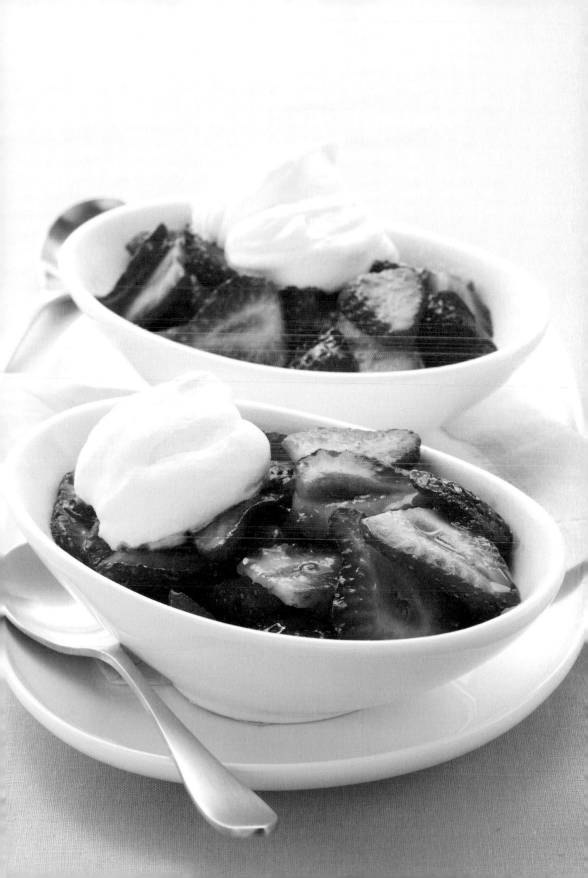

Sweet Potato Pudding

Since sweet potatoes are packed with natural sugar, this recipe requires just a bit of honey. Speed prep time by using the sweet potato you batch-cooked earlier in the week.

PREP: 15 minutes
COOK: 25 minutes
TOTAL TIME: 40 minutes
MAKES: 6 servings

Resistant Starch:

1.7 g

Cooking spray
2 large eggs
¼ cup honey, divided
¼ cup 1% low-fat milk
1 slice whole-wheat bread, crusts removed
2 cups mashed baked sweet potato
1 teaspoon vanilla extract
½ teaspoon ground cinnamon
¼ teaspoon ground allspice
2 tablespoons chopped pecans
2 tablespoons chopped crystallized ginger
¼ cup low-fat Greek yogurt

1. Preheat oven to 350°. Coat a 1½-quart baking dish with cooking spray.

2. Combine eggs, 3 tablespoons honey, milk, and bread in a large bowl. Beat with a mixer at medium speed until smooth. Add sweet potato, vanilla, cinnamon, and allspice; beat until smooth. Pour mixture into prepared baking dish. Sprinkle pecans and ginger over top. Bake at 350° for 25 minutes or until pudding is set and slightly puffy. (It will sink slightly as it cools.)

3. While pudding bakes, combine yogurt and remaining 1 tablespoon honey; stir until smooth. Divide pudding among 4 serving bowls; top each serving evenly with yogurt mixture.

Serving size: ½ cup pudding and 2 teaspoons topping | Calories 200; Fat 4g (sat 1g, mono 2g, poly 1g); Cholesterol 70mg; Protein 6g; Carbohydrate 38g; Sugars 20g; Fiber 3g; RS 1.7g; Sodium 95mg

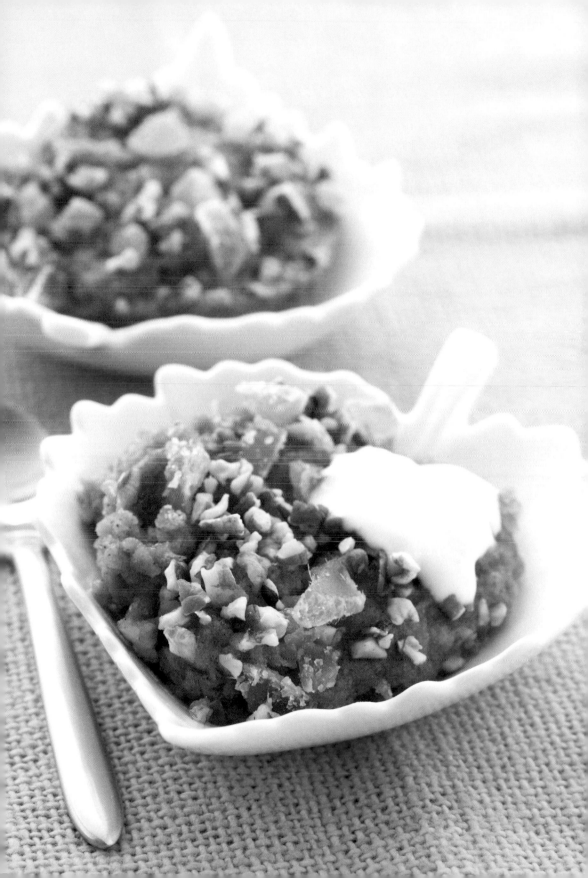

Raspberries with Chocolate Yogurt Mousse

Cocoa powder adds MUFAs, the yogurt is rich in CLA, and the raspberries pack plenty of fiber to make this a guilt-free treat.

PREP: 5 minutes
TOTAL TIME: 5 minutes
MAKES: 1 serving

> ½ **cup plain low–fat Greek yogurt**
> 1 **tablespoon unsweetened cocoa**
> 1 **tablespoon honey**
> ¼ **cup fresh raspberries**

1. Combine yogurt, cocoa, and honey in a serving bowl. Stir until blended. Top with raspberries.

Serving size: ½ cup yogurt and ¼ cup berries | Calories 170; Fat 3g (sat 2g, mono 0g, poly 0g); Cholesterol 10mg; Protein 11g; Carbohydrate 29g; Sugars 23g; Fiber 4g; RS 0g; Sodium 40mg

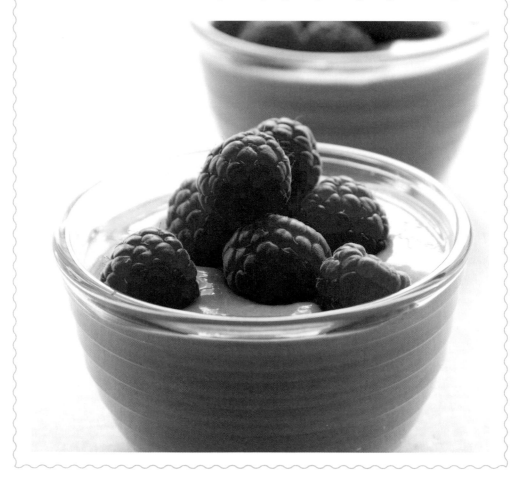

CARBLOVERS SMART RECIPE SWAPS

You know how some cookbooks teach you "makeover" techniques that turn an unhealthy recipe into a healthy one? The same principle applies here, but instead we show you how to "carb it up." It's fun to get creative and put a *CarbLovers* stamp on all of your personal recipes.

SWAP THIS OUT	SWAP THIS IN
Store-bought croutons	Toasted rye, pumpernickel, or sourdough bread; roasted potato cubes; baked polenta cubes
White rice	Brown rice
All-purpose flour	Whole-wheat flour: Replace up to one-third of all-purpose flour with regular whole-wheat flour and up to half with whole-wheat pastry flour.
White pasta	Whole-grain or fiber-fortified pasta
Mayonnaise (for spreads and dips)	Hummus, mashed avocado, low-fat Greek or regular yogurt, mashed white beans, pureed low-fat cottage cheese, pureed sweet potato, pureed green peas, or skordalia (page 175)
Breadcrumbs (for coating meat and fish)	Crumbled potato chips, cornflakes, puffed-wheat cereal, or crushed nuts
Butter or shortening	Mashed banana or dates. Start out by swapping half the butter or shortening for the same amount of mashed fruit. You might have to decrease other liquid ingredients in the recipe to get it just right.
Ground beef	Substitute beans for up to half of the ground beef in a recipe.

"I Lost Weight on CarbLovers"

BEFORE

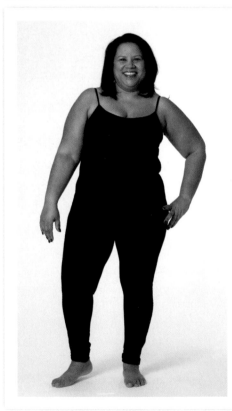

LUCY PASTRANA

Age: 45

Height: 5'6"

Weight before: 234

Weight after: 208

Pounds lost: 26

Biggest success moment:
The day my son came home with
18 Dunkin' Donuts! The old me would
have eaten one; the new me chose a
banana and almond butter.

Biggest challenge: Overeating
before my period. I crave sweets for
an entire week!

Favorite recipe: Fish Tacos with
Sesame-Ginger Slaw (page 172). The
creamy slaw makes it taste like takeout!

AFTER

I started *CarbLovers* because I wanted to weigh less than 200 pounds again. My weight has yo-yoed my entire life, from 150 pounds 23 years ago, just before I got married, to 250 pounds, after a tough year recently. I've tried Slim-Fast, Atkins, even the "cabbage soup" diet, but nothing helped. Within a month of beginning *CarbLovers,* I was introduced to whole-grain foods I'd never tried, like brown rice and cornmeal. These ingredients eased my cravings. I realized the lack of fiber in my usual snack fare—chips, donuts, or cookies— was making me eat way more sugar and sodium.

The most surprising part of this diet was the increase in my energy. I started taking an hour-long Zumba class after work. Before, I'd be exhausted after the class, eat a big snack, and fall asleep by 9:30. Now, dinner keeps me full, and I have no problem staying up until 11 cleaning my kitchen and reading. I feel like I'm drinking a cup of coffee!

CarbLovers taught me that as long as I have the right combination of vegetables, protein, and Resistant Starch, I won't feel hungry. And it can be on my terms. I created an alternative to the Zucchini & Potato Scramble with Bacon (page 137) by mixing sweet potato, bits of pork loin, egg whites, and spinach. Bottom line: At this point, I don't look at this diet as having a beginning, middle, and end. I see it as indulging in the healthy stuff for life. With only 8 pounds left to go, I'm confident I'll be less than 200 pounds by my 46th birthday!

Chapter 8

Reach Your *CarbLovers* Goal FASTER

YOU'RE FOUR WEEKS into *The CarbLovers Diet,* and it's time to reflect on your many successes. Chances are your pants are a lot looser. You're glowing (have you been getting compliments on your clear skin, bright eyes, and shiny hair? It's probably those carbs). Your mood is good—you feel less stressed, more energized than you have in years. Rather than obsessing over how little or how much you're eating, you're in a regular meal groove, enjoying the flavor, texture, and just plain yumminess of your favorite foods. Best of all, *you've lost up to 12 pounds.* If that's your final goal weight, congratulations! You can skip these pages and go directly to Chapter 10 for advice on maintaining your weight loss forever.

But if you want to lose 15, 35, even 100 or more pounds—here are two things I want you to do:

■ Continue the 21-Day *CarbLovers* Immersion Plan, but cut out one snack;

■ Follow the Get-to-Goal Strategies below. These simple tricks will help you lose weight even faster by zapping a few hundred extra calories a day. Try to incorporate at least two or even more of these into your life to really get the scale moving. Finally, only choose those strategies that you can actually stick with. Hate green tea or just can't make time for 8 hours of sleep a night? Do something else that you can commit to!

9 GET-TO-GOAL STRATEGIES THAT REALLY WORK

1. Automate eating.

Some people can lose weight while enjoying lots of variety in their food choices, while others discover that variety only stimulates their appetite. Frances Largeman-Roth, RD, calls this the "buffet effect" (you know, where you just...can't...stop eating because there are so many options?). There's some evidence that backs up this theory: When researchers at The University of Illinois at Urbana-Champaign offered study participants M&Ms in 10 different colors, they gobbled up 77 percent more candy than when offered just seven colors. In another study done by the same researchers, participants consumed 55 percent more jelly beans when they were offered 24 varieties of flavors versus only 6 varieties.[1] If you suspect too many different "tastes" makes you hungrier, try this: Instead of eating seven different breakfasts, lunches, dinners, and snacks each week, you may want to try alternating among just two or three of them. Dieters who have tried it say they actually appreciate having to make fewer decisions and feel fuller faster.

2. Control portions with frozen meals.

Replacing two or more dinners a week with frozen meals can be helpful when it comes to portion control: Since these kinds of meals are already portioned for you, there's no guesswork—and no chance you'll be tempted to have seconds or thirds. Use the list of recommended dinners on page 268 as a guide.

3. Cool your food.

If you enjoyed cold pizza or spaghetti for breakfast in college, now's a good time to get back in the habit. Cold foods are thought to help you to burn more fat and fill up on fewer calories. Cooking actually reduces the amount of Resistant Starch in a food because it causes the starch to absorb water and swell, breaking up the starch and making it more digestible. As a food cools, however, the starch recrystallizes back into Resistant Starch. This is why a cold boiled potato has twice as much Resistant Starch as a hot one. Eating cold, high-Resistant Starch foods may fill you up faster, so you don't need to eat everything on your plate. It will also provide you with an extra metabolism boost.[2]

4. Choose less-ripe fruit.

As fruit ripens, starch turns into sugar. This is why a green banana has 12.5 grams of Resistant Starch, whereas a ripe one has just 4.7 grams. Bottom line: The less ripe your fruit, the more Resistant Starch it will contain—and the more fat you'll burn.

5. Cook al dente.

The more a food is cooked, the more water the starch absorbs, causing the starch to become more digestible (which may hinder weight loss). This is why al dente foods are thought to offer you more slimming Resistant Starch than foods that have been cooked into limpness.[3]

6. Swap pepper for salt.

You know how you feel hot after a spicy meal? You're burning fat thanks to *capsaicin*, a substance in chile peppers that speeds metabolism. Some recipes in Chapter 7 contain cayenne and other hot spices, but if you want to boost your weight loss even more, try sprinkling a little red pepper on whatever you want.

7. Sip more green tea.

I hope you're already sipping my tried-and-true tea-based Fat-Flushing Cocktail on page 64. If not, consider this: Green tea packs two key metabolism boosters, and more tea could equal bigger weight loss. In one study, participants who consumed caffeinated green tea daily continued to lose weight after four weeks, whereas study participants who did not have the drink had significant weight regain. Other research has found that drinking a cup of green tea before your workout can increase your fat-burning during it. Very high amounts of green tea (the amount in several cups) has been shown to boost fat-burning up to 17 percent.[4,5]

8. Sleep an extra hour every night.

You really can sleep your way to a smaller waistline, and an hour or two more zzzs can make all the difference. When you don't get enough sleep, levels of the hunger hormone ghrelin rise and the satiety hormone leptin dips. This makes your body pile on belly fat, and it also makes you feel hungry, sluggish, and stressed. In fact, a study at Walter Reed Army Medical Center in Washington, DC, found that people who slept fewer than 6 hours a night tended to weigh more than people who slept more—even though these sleep skimpers walked an extra 1.5 miles a day. And a Harvard study of more than 68,000 women determined that those who slept 5 hours or less a night gained 2.5 pounds more over a 16-year period than women who regularly slept 7 hours or more.[6,7]

9. Exercise (some).

You don't have to pump iron or run 5 miles a day to succeed on *CarbLovers*. But exercise will help you lose weight more quickly, and you'll feel great doing it, too. Now is the perfect time to get back into shape with The *CarbLovers* Workout on page 239.[8] It's an optional routine that combines strength-training and cardio, burning loads of calories in under 20 minutes! If that's too much structure for you, then try these oldies but goodies: Take the stairs instead of the elevator, consider walking or biking to work rather than driving, or spend an afternoon walking with friends or your family instead of doing errands by car.

Your energy on carbs

Carbs prevent fatigue in two ways. They keep muscle glycogen levels stocked to capacity, which gives you more energy during workouts. What's more, high-Resistant Starch carbs help your body burn fat more efficiently, so you stay energized longer.

Ask the carb pro

Frances Largeman-Roth, RD

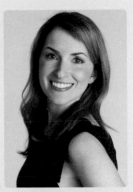

Q. Will exercising while on *CarbLovers* make me binge—and not lose weight?

A. No. Bottom line is that even if you feel hungrier after a workout, you're still probably burning more calories than you take in. Researchers recently studied 12 people, tracking their energy expenditure and food intake for 16 days. The participants were hungrier after they exercised, but they only compensated (by eating) for about 30 percent of the calories burned. In other words, 70 percent of the calories they burned during exercise stayed burned. An Australian study found that exercising made study participants feel hungrier just before meals, but they felt satisfied more quickly when they did eat. So you'll always be ahead of the game if you exercise!

"I Lost Weight on CarbLovers"

BEFORE

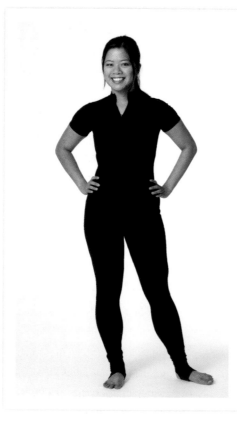

SERENA TONG

Age: 28

Height: 5'5"

Weight before: 137

Weight after: 127

Pounds lost: 10

Biggest success moment: When I got on the scale and saw a sustained weight loss every week. When I had done crash diets before, I'd yo-yo, but I knew this diet was working because I consistently lost every week.

Biggest challenge: Ending my addiction to fast food. *CarbLovers* taught me to make quick meals.

Favorite recipe: Bacon, Pear & Gorgonzola Pizza (page 194). It tasted like what comes out of a delivery box!

AFTER

I started CarbLovers because I was getting married, and I wanted to look my best in my curve-hugging, trumpet-style gown. But I needed to find a diet that I could sustain beyond my honeymoon. When I started *The CarbLovers Diet*, "starch" was a four-letter word. I've tried low-carb diets, like South Beach, before, and I kept the weight off for a month but always gained it back.

During the first phase of *CarbLovers*, it took commitment to buy the whole foods listed on the recipes and actually cook. At first, I relied mainly on portion control. Instead of eating two pieces of whole-wheat toast each morning, I'd swap one of those for an egg or other type of lean protein. Eventually I realized many of the meals were simple enough for me to cook for dinner after a long day's work. The biggest surprise on the diet was how full I felt when I began adding Resistant Starch-filled foods. Even during the first few weeks, I realized I could eat less food and still be as full. It was hard to stress-eat when I was so full!

And unlike other diets, there was a lot of real food, rather than those processed, fat-free snacks that can set you up for an afternoon meltdown. As the diet progressed, I learned that if I allowed an hour or two on Sunday night, I could prepare all my lunches for the week. Knowing that I had a stash of healthy lunches made me less stressed.

CarbLovers has taught me that eating the right types of carbohydrates is a good thing for my body. Finally, I've found a diet that controls my stress-eating, doesn't make me feel deprived, and has gotten me back to my "happy weight."

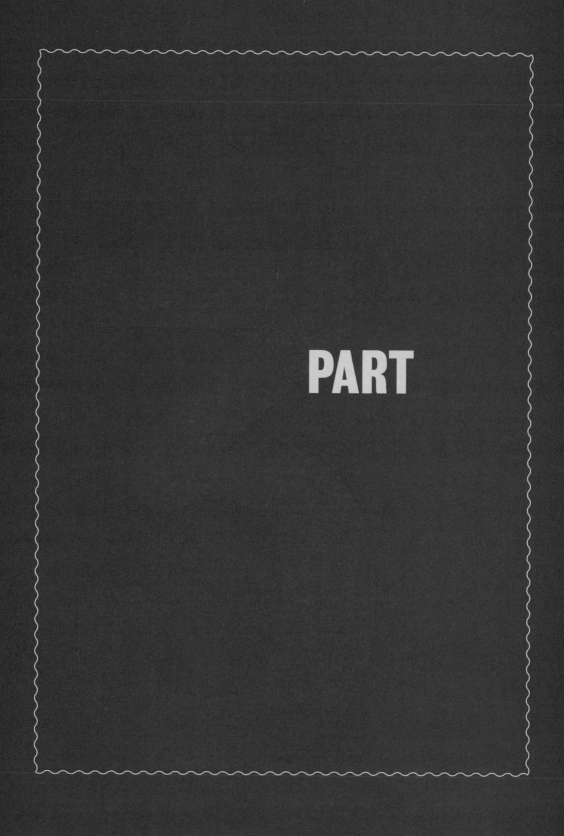

PART

Eat Carbs, Stay Slim— For Life!

Chapter 9

The
CarbLovers
Workout

GOOD NEWS: You don't have to pump iron or run marathons to succeed on *The CarbLovers Diet.* But exercise will help you lose weight more quickly (and keep it off), and you'll feel great doing it, too. That's because a diet rich in Resistant Starch and other carb foods fuels your muscles, speeds your metabolism, and makes your energy soar! This three-part, full-body routine takes less than 30 minutes, and you can do it at home or at the gym. You'll burn nearly 900 extra calories a week, plus trim up to 3 inches a month from your belly, hips, and thighs! **NOTE: Please get clearance from your doctor before starting The *CarbLovers* Workout, especially if you've been inactive for a while.**

1. *CARBLOVERS* SUPER TONE-UP!

Doing this all-over strength workout twice a week gets you extra benefits: Each move is a "compound" exercise, meaning it targets multiple muscle groups.

Workout Planner

Do these moves with dumbbells, a sturdy bench or step, a mat, and a stability ball. Here's a sample schedule; feel free to skip a day here and there.

Monday: Cardio Interval Workout
Tuesday: *CarbLovers* **Super Tone-Up!**
Wednesday: Cardio Interval Workout
Thursday: Firm Your Belly Routine
Friday: Cardio Interval Workout
Saturday: *CarbLovers* **Super Tone-Up!**
Sunday: Cardio Interval Workout

Squat To Overhead Press

for quadriceps, hamstrings, butt, abs, shoulders

A. Stand with feet shoulder-width apart, elbows bent, a 5-pound weight in each hand at shoulder height, palms forward. Lower into a squat (don't let knees go past toes); hold for a moment.

B. Push through heels to stand up, pressing weights overhead. Return to starting position. Do 3 sets of 15 reps.

Single-Leg Dumbbell Row

for back, shoulders, biceps, abs, quadriceps, hamstrings, butt

A. Stand holding a 5- to 10-pound weight in right hand. Hinge forward so back is flat and almost parallel to floor; rest left hand on a chair or low shelf for support. Extend right arm toward floor, palm facing in; lift straight right leg behind you so body forms a T.

B. Slowly bend right elbow and draw weight up until elbow is even with torso; hold for a moment, and then lower weight. Do 15 reps, and then switch sides and repeat. Do 3 sets.

Step-Up With Bicep Curl
for quadriceps, hamstrings, butt, abs, biceps

A. Stand with right foot on a sturdy bench or step, with a 5-pound weight in each hand.

B. With weight on right foot, lift to standing on the step, left thigh raised so it's parallel to floor; at the same time, curl weights up toward shoulders. Return to starting position. Do 15 reps, and then switch sides and repeat. Do 3 sets.

Superman
for back, butt

Lie face down with arms and legs extended, toes pointed, palms down. Inhale while raising arms and legs as high as you can; pause, and then exhale while slowly returning to starting position. Do 3 sets of 15 reps.

Dolphin Plank
for back, abs, shoulders

A. Lie face down with toes tucked. Keeping forearms on floor, pull belly button in toward spine and raise hips to come into low plank position.

B. Inhale while lifting hips further so body forms an inverted V; pause, and then slowly return to starting position. Do 3 sets of 15 reps.

Curtsy Lunge
for hips, butt, quadriceps, hamstrings, abs

Stand with feet hip-width apart, hands on hips. Take a giant step diagonally back with left foot and cross it behind your right; bend knees (as if curtsying) as you reach your left hand toward floor on the outside of your right foot. Return to starting position. Do 15 reps, and then switch sides and repeat. Do 3 sets.

2. FIRM YOUR BELLY ROUTINE

Completing this belly-focused set will help you get flatter abs in no time. It's fine to do this series on the same day as you do the all-over tone-up routine, too.

Crunch 'n' Reach

A. Lie with your shoulder blades, back, and hips on a stability ball, knees shoulder-width apart and bent to 90 degrees, feet on the floor. Extend your arms overhead.

B. Draw your lower abdomen in toward your spine. Slowly raise your arms above your shoulders while lifting your chest so that both shoulder blades and your upper back come off the ball. Hold for 3 seconds, and then return to starting position. That's 1 rep. Do 3 sets of 15 reps.

Twisting Knee Crunch

A. Lie on your back on a stability ball with feet hip-distance apart on the floor and knees bent to 90 degrees. Bring your left hand behind your head and your right fingertips to the floor for balance. Brace your core and lift your right foot off the floor. Extend your right leg, foot flexed.

B. Crunch up, twisting your left shoulder and rib cage toward your right knee while simultaneously stretching your left leg straight (keep your foot on the floor). Return to starting position (right leg lifted, left leg bent). That's 1 rep. Do 15 reps, and then switch sides and repeat. Do 3 sets.

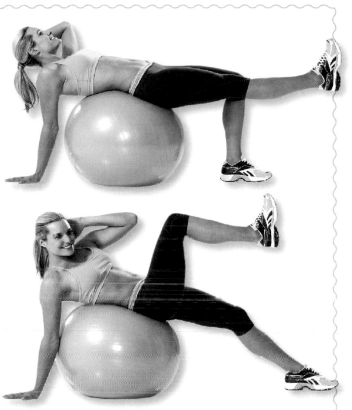

Stir the Pot

Kneel in front of a stability ball with your forearms and elbows on the ball, hands clasped. Roll the ball forward until your legs are extended and your body is in plank position, toes tucked. Your shoulders should be stacked directly above your elbows, chest lifted off the ball, and neck in line with your spine. Brace your abs, and make small circles to the right with your forearms, as if stirring a pot. Do 15 reps, and then repeat, making circles to the left. Do 3 sets.

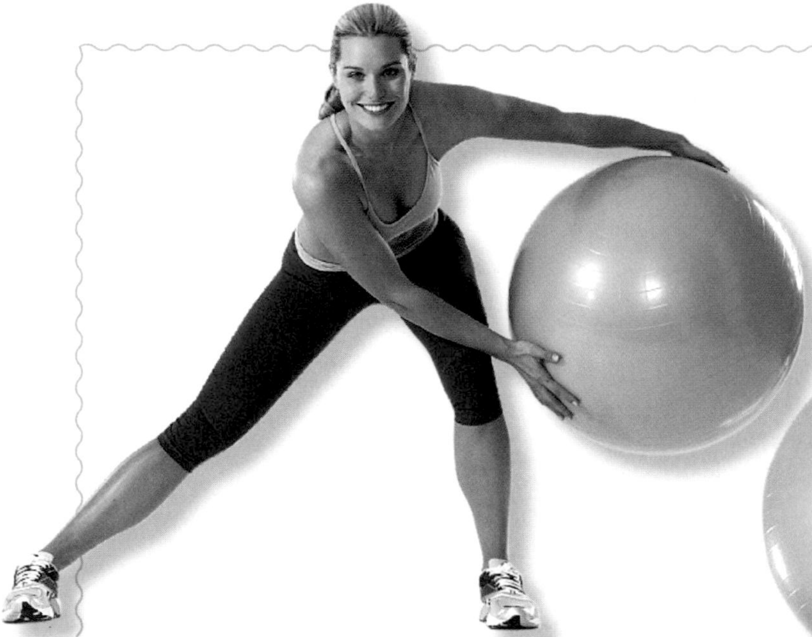

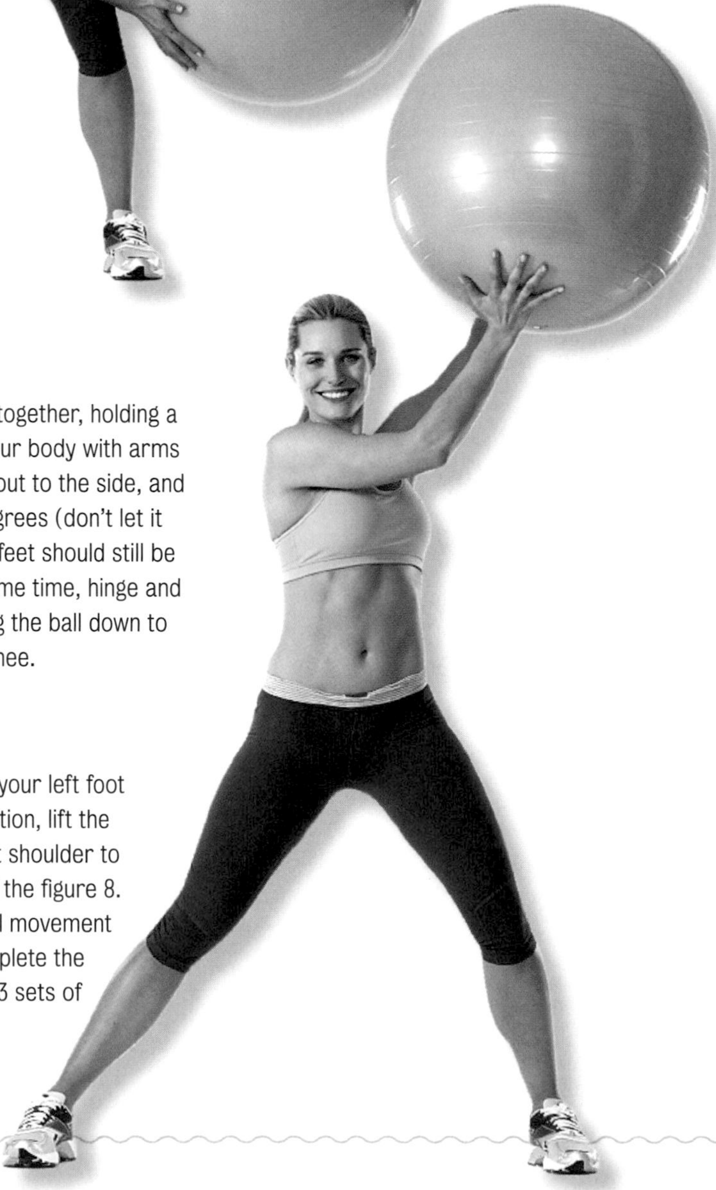

Figure 8 Lunge

A. Stand with your feet together, holding a stability ball in front of your body with arms bent. Step your left foot out to the side, and bend your knee to 90 degrees (don't let it go past your toes); both feet should still be facing forward. At the same time, hinge and twist at your hips to bring the ball down to the outside of your left knee.

B. As you push off with your left foot to return to starting position, lift the ball up and over your left shoulder to complete the first half of the figure 8. Repeat the lunge and ball movement on the other side to complete the figure 8; that's 1 rep. Do 3 sets of 15 reps.

3. BLAST FAT & CALORIES CARDIO INTERVAL WORKOUT:

Burn fat and stoke your metabolism by doing one of these interval workouts for 35 minutes four times per week. The intensity levels are based on a scale of 1 to 10, where 1 is not much effort and 10 is pushing as hard as you can.

Outdoor walking workout:
- Walk at an intensity of 3 to 4 for 4 minutes to warm up.
- Pick up your pace for 3 minutes so you're working at a 6 to 7.
- Crank your pace up to an 8 for 2 minutes. Take shorter, faster steps, drive your bent elbows back, and let your hips move.
- Repeat steps 2 and 3 four more times.

Treadmill workout:
- Walk at a moderate pace with no incline (an intensity of 3 to 4) for 4 minutes to warm up.
- Pick up your speed to a 6 to 7 for 3 minutes.
- Rev up your pace to an 8, and increase the incline to 2 for 2 minutes.
- Repeat steps 2 and 3 four more times.

Elliptical workout:
- Use light resistance with a medium ramp (for an intensity of 3 to 4) for 4 minutes to warm up.
- Keeping light resistance, raise ramp to high for 3 minutes, aiming for an intensity of 6 to 7.
- Lower ramp and increase resistance; work at a challenging pace (about an 8) for 2 minutes.
- Repeat steps 2 and 3 four more times.

Bike workout (outdoor or indoor):
- Pedal at medium (an intensity of 3 to 4) for 4 minutes to warm up.
- Increase your speed and/or resistance to moderate intensity (6 to 7) for 3 minutes.
- Up your intensity to an 8 for 2 minutes.
- Repeat steps 2 and 3 four more times.

"I Lost Weight on *CarbLovers*"

BEFORE

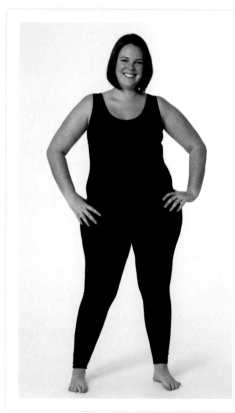

MELISSA THOMAS

Age: 27

Height: 5'8"

Weight before: 212

Weight after: 197

Pounds lost: 15

Biggest success moment: Getting to a healthy weight so I can be a healthy mom in the future.

Biggest challenge: Even with the flexibility of *CarbLovers*, there were still times I faced temptation. To dodge it, I tell myself how much exercise I'll have to do if I give in—like, "it takes me an hour to burn off a candy bar"—and most of the time it's just not worth it.

Favorite recipe: Chocolate-Dipped Banana Bites (page 212) and Dark Chocolate & Oat Clusters (page 213)!

AFTER

My husband and I hope to have a baby soon, and I want to lose weight before getting pregnant. Last year I tried and failed on two different diets: One was all about counting points (so tedious). The other was super-strict: Some days I couldn't have protein, other days I couldn't have cooked veggies, and on other days I couldn't have carbs. Bleah. Both diets had too many restrictions. Each time, I ended up quitting, regaining the weight I'd lost, and going back to my old size 16-18 clothes.

I hoped *CarbLovers* would address the problem I had with other diets—and it did! It is simple, flexible, and allows me to eat anything and everything I want, even chips, chocolate, and olives. When I saw the plan, I was like, "Wow...I can have olives?" There's no one telling me I can't have something!

The recipes were easy to adapt, too. After I learned about how important Resistant Starches are, I started using them in my own recipes. For example, I added corn and black beans to my favorite turkey burger recipe.

Best of all, I'm getting the weight-loss results I want! I lost 4 pounds during the first week, and after 10 weeks I lost 15 pounds. I've got about 22 pounds to go until I reach my goal—I'm definitely sticking with *CarbLovers!*

Chapter 10

CarbLovers
for Life!

YOU'VE REACHED YOUR GOAL WEIGHT, and you're feeling absolutely amazing. You're also probably feeling just a little bit nervous. That's because you've lost weight before, but then you gained back every pound, plus a few extra. NOT THIS TIME. *CarbLovers* was designed to be the diet that finally allows you to achieve permanent weight loss. And it really will work. Here's why: On *CarbLovers*, you didn't cut out anything to lose the weight, so you don't have any foods or food groups to add back in. (We didn't even ask you to give up potato chips or wine or chocolate!) Nothing has been off limits during the diet, so there's no risk of you pigging out on foods you've been craving.

What's more, the dietitians who created *CarbLovers* found a sneaky way to make sure you would stay as thin as you are today. The new you has been eating the right foods in the right portions all along. Phase 2 of *The CarbLovers Diet* had you eating 1,600 calories (and your daily target of Resistant Starch-rich foods) a day, and if you're at your goal now, that's exactly the right amount to help you maintain your new smaller self.

Of course, if your pants feel a little too snug again, go right back to Chapter 8 for quick weight-loss strategies. And if you're one of those rare, lucky people who can't stop losing weight while enjoying all the carbs you want, then go ahead— eat an extra snack or allow yourself slightly bigger portions.

Many people make the mistake of eating more or changing things up once they reach their weight-loss goal. But here's the deal: Your metabolism slows down as your body gets lighter. So you can't go back to eating what it took to maintain your weight at, say, 160 pounds—now that you weigh 130.

At the same time, now that you've tasted real weight-loss success, it's time to expand your horizons. There are steps you need to take over the next few weeks, months, even years to make a complete transition from following *The CarbLovers Diet* to living the *CarbLovers* Life. But the rules are straightforward and easy-to-follow (and you've been practicing). If you follow them, you'll learn to make smart food choices automatically at your book club, on vacation, even at your Thanksgiving table.

Ask the carb pro

Frances Largeman-Roth, RD

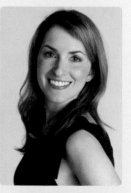

Q. How can I stay on track with *CarbLovers* when I'm juggling work, kids, laundry...?

A. Use the power of the Post-It to keep Resistant Starch in mind. Put notes on your fridge, mirror, dashboard, etc., with messages like "Beans are Beautiful" and "Bananas = Bikini Body."

4 *CARBLOVERS* RULES
IN THE KITCHEN

1. Make at least **one** meal a day that includes all of these:

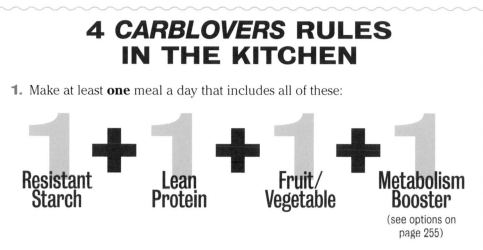

Resistant Starch	Lean Protein	Fruit/ Vegetable	Metabolism Booster

(see options on
page 255)

If you can't include a metabolism booster or a protein at a meal, double your serving of Resistant Starch in order to compensate. Otherwise you'll end up hungry. For the perfect *CarbLovers* portions, see the chart on pages 254–255.

2. When choosing among grains and starches, always choose Resistant Starch (see the charts on pages 254 and 272) or high-fiber carbs (see the chart on page 273) over highly refined starches such as regular pasta (made from refined flour), white rice, white bread, and low-fiber breakfast cereals.

3. Choose high-performance fats such as MUFAs and omega-3s (for a list, see pages 274–275). Specifically, we're talking about avocados, olives and olive oil, fatty fish such as anchovies and salmon, peanuts, seeds and nuts, and coconut products. Use olive oil on salads instead of other cooking oils on salads. Use guacamole or hummus as a sandwich spread in place of butter and mayo.

4. When adding flavor to various dishes, consider using a metabolism booster, such as cayenne pepper, vinegar, or anchovy paste.

CARBLOVERS PORTION SIZES

HIGH–RESISTANT STARCH CHOICES
(150 calories)
1 large banana
¾ cup barley
½ cup beans
2 slices whole-grain bread (1-ounce slices)
1 whole-wheat English muffin
1 ounce corn tortilla chips
1¼ cups cornflakes
2½ cups puffed wheat
⅔ cup cooked polenta
4 crispbread crackers
½ cup cooked lentils
¾ cup cooked millet
¾ cup cooked brown rice
½ cup oatmeal, uncooked (1 cup cooked)
1 cup cooked whole-wheat pasta
1 cup cooked peas
2 small pitas
¾ cup plantain
3 cups popped popcorn
1 ounce potato chips
1 small potato, baked
1 cup potatoes, cooked and cooled
2 (6-inch) tortillas
1 cup cooked cubed yams

LEAN PROTEIN CHOICES (cooked portion)
(150 calories)
3 ounces skinless poultry
3 ounces fish (especially salmon)
2 ounces lean beef
½ cup edamame
¾ cup tofu
1 cup soy crumbles
2 eggs

PRODUCE

Vegetables

(unlimited, no portion control needed!)

Artichokes
Asparagus
Bean sprouts
Bok choy
Broccoli
Brussels sprouts
Cabbage
Carrots
Cauliflower
Celery
Collard greens
Cucumbers
Dark green leafy lettuce
Eggplant
Green or red bell peppers
Iceberg lettuce
Kale
Mesclun
Mushrooms
Mustard greens
Okra
Onions
Romaine lettuce
Spinach
Tomatoes
Turnip greens
Watercress
Wax beans
Zucchini

Fruit

Any medium whole fruit
1 cup berries or sliced fruit

METABOLISM-BOOSTING CHOICES

(100 calories or less)

1 tbsp olive oil
⅛ cup nuts or seeds
1 tbsp peanut butter
1 tbsp almond butter
3 tbsp coconut milk
⅓ cup shredded coconut
¼ bar chocolate
2 tbsp flaxseeds or flaxseed meal
¾ cup low-fat yogurt
1 slice low-fat cheese
1 cup low-fat milk
½ cup low-fat soft cheese (ricotta, cottage, etc)
1 small whole fruit
1 cup sliced fruit
½ cup dried fruit

SCORE A PERFECT RS 10

All the meals in *The CarbLovers Diet* add up to *at least* 10 grams of fat-flushing Resistant Starch a day. But it's easy to get the Resistant Starch you need on your own! Just use the list of high-Resistant Starch carbs on page 254 along with the nutritional info with the *CarbLovers* recipes to count RS grams and make sure your own menu adds up to a slimmer you. Here's a quick RS cheat sheet.

BREAKFAST CARBS +	LUNCH CARBS +	DINNER CARBS =	10+ GRAMS OF RESISTANT STARCH PER DAY
1 banana (4.7 g) in a smoothie	½ cup white beans (3.8 g)	1 serving whole grain pasta (2 g)	10.5 g
1 banana (4.7 g) with oatmeal (0.5g)	Sandwich on rye bread (1.8 g)	½ cup brown rice (1.7g) with ½ cup black beans (1.5 g)	10.2 g
Cornflakes (0.9 g) with banana (4.7 g)	Ham, Sliced Pear & Swiss Sandwich (2.6 g)	½ cup barley (1.9 g)	10.1 g
Banana & Almond Butter Toast (5.6 g)	Black Bean & Zucchini Quesadillas (4.7 g)	Baked potato (1.4 g)	11.7g
Puffed wheat cereal (0.9 g)	Greek Lentil Soup with Toasted Pita (5.3 g)	Barley Risotto Primavera (4.1 g)	10.3 g
Breakfast Barley with Banana & Sunflower Seeds (7.6 g)	Sandwich on pumpernickel bread (2.6 g) with 1 ounce potato chips (1 g)	½ cup millet (1.5 g)	12.7 g
Apple & Almond Muesli (4.6 g)	Potato salad (2.3 g) over greens with rye crackers (0.8 g)	Bistro-Style Sirloin with New Potatoes (2.3 g)	10 g
Blueberry Oat Pancakes with Maple Yogurt (4.6 g)	Mediterranean Pasta Salad (2.4 g)	Black Bean Tacos (4.7 g)	11 g

Use Resistant Starch
ingredients like these
to build your own
CarbLovers meals!

4 STEPS TO A *CARBLOVERS* RESTAURANT MEAL

1. Skip the entree. Instead, have two sides and one appetizer (see our Clip & Carry cheat sheet on the next page). That's dinner. Main courses at most restaurants offer more food than any normal human being should be eating and will probably come in at half your total calorie count for the day. By following these "side" rules, you'll stick to your diet and never feel hungry!

2. Order a *CarbLovers* starch side dish. Always swap empty-carbs side dishes (refined bread, pasta, rice) for Resistant Starch carbs, like corn and brown rice (use the lists on pages 254 and 272). If a Resistant Starch carb is not available, go for high-fiber carbs as a second option (see page 273 for a list). And take your carbs naked. That means no sauce or butter. Have baked potatoes instead of scalloped, brown rice instead of rice pilaf, and plain bread instead of buttered.

3. Combine your Resistant Starch side dish with a vegetable, either as a side dish (like steamed broccoli) or as a small salad. (No fattening add-ons like sour cream or fried onions!)

4. Add an appetizer. Good options include: shrimp cocktail ceviche, black bean soup, turkey chili, and shrimp or chicken kabobs. Order appetizers baked, grilled, broiled, or steamed; avoid anything that's breaded and fried, because they may not be prepared with healthy fats.

Congratulations! Start enjoying your new carb-filled life!

I am absolutely thrilled that you've embraced carbs (and *CarbLovers*), lost all the weight you wanted, and have reached your goal (or soon will)…for good. Please send me an update on your fabulous new life and share photos of yourself before you started *CarbLovers* and how you look today at **carblovers@health.com!**

Before, you were probably obsessed with dieting: *Can I resist that doughnut? I'm not sure if I should eat that slice of bread. I can't have pasta!* But now, all the dieting and the hunger has finally ended, and you can allow something else to become the center of your life. The best news of all: Now that you're eating in a way that really nourishes your whole self, you have an untapped reservoir of energy that you can apply to the rest of your life. Get out there, and enjoy every bite of it.

Clip & Carry
The *CarbLovers* Diet
Restaurant Cheat Sheet

American

(suggested menu items to mix and match)
Baked potato + steamed asparagus + shrimp cocktail
Baked sweet potato + steamed broccoli + steak skewers

Italian

(suggested menu items to mix and match)
Whole-grain roll + basic house salad with light vinaigrette + steamed mussels
Sliced whole-wheat baguette + basic house salad with light vinaigrette + grilled calamari

Indian

(suggested menu items to mix and match)
Brown rice + vegetable kabobs + chicken tikka (marinated chicken)
Roti (whole-wheat bread) + vegetable kabobs + dahl (lentil stew)

Chinese/Asian

(suggested menu items to mix and match)
Brown rice + garlic snap peas + steamed shrimp dumplings
Brown rice + spicy green beans + chicken lettuce wraps

Mediterranean

(suggested menu items to mix and match)
Whole-grain pita + basic Greek salad (tomato, cucumber, onion, olives,
    green bell pepper—easy on the Feta & dressing) + hummus
Skordalia (potato-garlic dip) + basic Greek salad (tomato, cucumber, onion,
    olives, green bell pepper—easy on the Feta & dressing) + chicken satay

Mexican

(suggested menu items to mix and match)
Tortilla chips (not fried) + salsa + black bean soup
Corn tortillas + fajita-style vegetables + fajita-style chicken or steak

"I Lost Weight on *CarbLovers*"

BEFORE

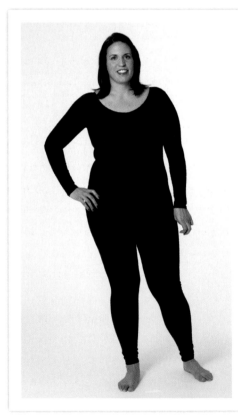

CARISSA PELLETIER

Age: 34

Height: 5'11"

Weight before: 218

Weight after: 204

Pounds lost: 14

Biggest success moment: I'm fitting comfortably into some clothes that I could only just squeeze into before.

Biggest challenge: Not being 100 percent supported by my friends and family who don't have to diet.

Favorite recipe: I LOVED both of the taco recipes—the Fish Tacos with Sesame-Ginger Slaw (page 172) and the Black Bean Tacos (page 104). They don't taste like diet food at all.

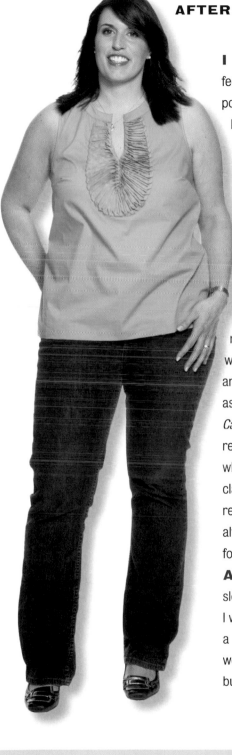

AFTER

I tried *CarbLovers* because I wasn't feeling good about my weight or myself. At 218 pounds (and creeping up), I reached a point where I was ready to do something about it. Other diets didn't give me enough food—I was hungry all the time. But *CarbLovers* put real food on the menu. The idea of making pasta, tacos, and desserts inspired me to restock my pantry and fridge and actually plan meals. Have you ever heard of anyone being excited about cooking on a diet? Well I was. The *CarbLovers* recipes were easy and delicious!

I wasn't surprised to lose 4 pounds in my first week—but I was surprised that I did it without starving myself! The wholesome carbs and Resistant Starch are as filling and satisfying as promised. Once I learned the principles of *CarbLovers*, I used them to tweak my own favorite recipes. For example, I cook with more whole-wheat pasta now—I use it to make linguine with clam sauce. I also changed the way I order in restaurants: I ask for more vegetables and always swap brown rice for white when we go for Chinese food.

After 12 weeks, my weight loss has slowed down, but I am a whole size smaller than I was when I first began *CarbLovers*. I'm planning a trip to Aruba in a few months, and with the weight I've lost, I'm going to reward myself by buying a new, smaller swimsuit for that trip!

Chapter 11

The *CarbLovers* Ultimate Eat-Out Guide

IN THIS CHAPTER, you'll get even more support to help you follow *The CarbLovers Diet* no matter where you are. Need to know what to order at a restaurant or a fast-food counter? It's here. Wish you could swap in a frozen meal for one of the recipe options given in Phase 1 and 2? Find great choices here. Want to know which brands of packaged foods are high in Resistant Starch, fiber, omega-3s, and other metabolism boosters—*without* having to read the fine print on every label? Done. You'll even find the right foods in the right portion sizes so you don't have to do the math yourself.

CarbLovers Restaurant Options

The following choices all contain at least one ingredient high in Resistant Starch as well as several other metabolism boosters. You can mix and match them, too. Pair any option that totals fewer than 300 calories with a medium piece of fruit.

RECOMMENDED BREAKFAST OPTIONS (PHASE 1 OR 2)

Food	Calories	Serving Size
Panera Strawberry Granola Parfait	280	8.25 oz
Au Bon Pain Apple Cinnamon Oatmeal	280	12 oz (medium)
Starbucks Apple Bran Muffin with Omega 3s & 7g Fiber	350	121g muffin
Dunkin' Donuts Ham, Egg White & Cheese on Wheat English Muffin	300	1 sandwich
Così Oatmeal	101	7.5 oz
Jamba Juice Fresh Banana Oatmeal	280	9.6 oz
Jamba Juice Blueberry & Blackberry Oatmeal	290	8.9 oz
Jamba Juice Coldbuster	240	16 fl oz
Jamba Juice Protein Berry Workout with Soy Protein	270	16 fl oz
Orange Julius Bananarilla	400	20 oz (medium)
Orange Julius Berry Banana Squeeze	270	20 oz
Subway Egg & Cheese Sandwich on 9-grain bread with egg white	320	1 6" sandwich
Subway Ham, Egg & Cheese Sandwich on 9-grain bread with egg white	350	1 6" sandwich

RECOMMENDED LUNCH AND DINNER OPTIONS (PHASE 1 OR 2)

These meals can all be eaten in the portion sizes in which they're sold, so you can enjoy everything on your plate. Mix and match them for lunch and dinner. Pair any option that's less than 300 calories with a small side salad or piece of fruit.

Food	Calories	Serving Size
Jamba Juice Chimichurri Chicken Wrap without sauce	410	1 wrap
Fazoli's Grilled Chicken Artichoke Salad	240	12.3 oz
Cosi Hummus & Veggie Sandwich	397	10.2 oz
P.F. Chang's Buddha's Feast steamed with a side of brown rice	210	9 oz lunch bowl
Wendy's Sour Cream & Chives Baked Potato	320	1 potato
Wendy's Small Chili with Side Salad	225	227g chili, 225g salad
Einstein Bros Traditional Potato Salad	355	½ cup
Einstein Bros Half Chicken Chipotle Salad	365	7.8 oz
Wendy's Southwest Taco Salad	400	1 salad
Subway Oven Roasted Chicken Sandwich on 9-grain wheat bread	310	1 6" sandwich
Subway Turkey Breast Sandwich on 9-grain wheat bread	280	1 6" sandwich
Subway Veggie Delite Sandwich on 9-grain wheat bread	230	1 6" sandwich

Your immunity on carbs

Consuming more Resistant Starch protects you from disease in two ways: It boosts disease-fighting bacteria in your digestive system by as much as 300 percent, which in turn crowds out the harmful kinds of bacteria that can cause digestive issues and the flu.

RECOMMENDED LUNCH AND DINNER OPTIONS (PHASE 2)

These options contain all the right ingredients, but they work best during Phase 2. The portions are too large for a single *CarbLovers* meal. Eat only ¾ of what you are served and save the rest to eat as a snack, or skip a snack for the day for servings that total more than 500 calories:

Food	Calories	Serving Size
Au Bon Pain Mayan Chicken Harvest Rice Bowl with Brown Rice	383	¾ of bowl
Au Bon Pain Spicy Tuna Sandwich	353	¾ of sandwich
Olive Garden Shrimp Primavera (lunch portion)	383	¾ of entree
Chili's "Guiltless Grill" Grilled Chicken Sandwich with Veggies	458	¾ of sandwich
Cosi Grilled Wild Alaskan Salmon Salad	343	¾ of salad
Cosi Tuscan Pesto Chicken Sandwich	383	¾ of sandwich
Panera Fuji Apple Chicken Salad	390	¾ of salad
Jamba Juice Grab-n-Go Greens and Grain Wrap	435 without sauce	¾ of wrap
Subway Tuna Sandwich on 9-grain wheat bread	398	¾ of 6" sandwich
Einstein Bros. California Chicken Wrap	473	¾ of wrap

CarbLovers Frozen Meals

These frozen meals all contain at least one high Resistant Starch ingredient. Swap them for any meal on The *CarbLovers* Plan.

RECOMMENDED BREAKFAST OPTIONS (PHASE 1 OR 2)

Serve any breakfast option that contains fewer than 250 calories (see asterisks*) along with a banana (preferred) or another piece of fruit.

Food	Calories	Serving Size
Jimmy Dean D-lights Turkey Bacon Bowl*	240	1
Aunt Jemima Sausage & Egg Scramble	300	1
Jimmy Dean D-lights Turkey Sausage Whole Grain Bagel	260	1
Bob Evans Hearty Blueberry Oatmeal Bowl*	240	1
Smart Ones Breakfast Quesadilla	220	1
Smart Ones Stuffed Breakfast Sandwich*	240	1
Amy's Breakfast Burrito*	250	1
Amy's Breakfast Scramble Wrap	380	1
Amy's Multi-Grain Hot Cereal Bowl*	190	1
Amy's Steel-Cut Oats Hot Cereal Bowl	220	1
Amy's Tofu Scramble	320	1
Aunt Jemima Great Starts Scrambled Eggs & Bacon with Hash Brown Potatoes	320	1
Lean Pockets Applewood Bacon, Egg, & Cheese	290	1
Bob Evans Cranberry Pecan Oatmeal Bowl	290	1
Fiber One Blueberry Muffins*	180	1
VitaMuffins Deep Chocolate (2)*	200	2
Vita Tops Banana Nut (2)*	200	2
Eggo Nutri-Grain Waffles (2)*	170	2

RECOMMENDED LUNCH AND DINNER OPTIONS (PHASE 1 OR 2)

Pair each lunch and dinner option with a small side salad and 2 tablespoons low-fat vinaigrette or steamed vegetables.

Food	Calories	Serving Size
Healthy Choice Oven Roasted Chicken	260	1
Healthy Choice Café Steamers Chicken Pesto Classico	320	1
Marie Callender's Honey Roasted Turkey	310	1
Kashi Lemongrass Coconut Chicken	300	1
Kashi Black Bean Mango	340	1
Kashi Ranchero Beans	340	1
Lean Cuisine Sun Dried Tomato Pesto Chicken	290	1
Lean Cuisine Ginger Garlic Stir Fry with Chicken	280	1
Lean Cuisine Salmon with Basil	220	1
Boston Market Oven Roasted Chicken	390	1
Amy's Black Bean Vegetable Enchilada	360	1
Amy's Mexican Tofu Scramble	400	1
Amy's Spinach Feta in a Pocket Sandwich	260	1
Amy's Vegetable Pie in a Pocket Sandwich	300	1
Amy's Bean & Rice Burrito	300	1
Amy's Black Bean Vegetable Burrito	290	1
Amy's Indian Samosa Wrap	250	1
Amy's Southwestern Burrito	300	1
Lean Pockets Whole Grain Turkey, Broccoli, and Cheese	260	1
Lean Pockets Whole Grain Grilled Chicken, Mushroom, and Spinach	250	1

CarbLovers Energy/Meal Bars

Food	Calories	Serving Size
Nutri-Grain Blueberry, Strawberry, or Blackberry Bar	130	1 bar
ExtendBar, any flavor (except Peanut Butter Crunch)	150	1 bar
Kashi TLC Raspberry Chocolate Fruit & Grain Bar	120	1 bar
Kashi TLC Pumpkin Pie Fruit & Grain Bar	120	1 bar
Kashi TLC Pumpkin Spice Flax or Honey Toasted 7-Grain Crunchy Granola Bars	170	1 bar
Kashi TLC Honey Almond Flax or Peanut Peanut Butter or Trail Mix Chewy Granola Bar	140	1 bar
Kashi TLC Cherry Dark Chocolate Chewy Granola Bar	120	1 bar
Fiber One Oats and Apple Streusel	130	1 bar
Fiber One Oats and Strawberry with Almonds	140	1 bar
Fiber One Oats and Peanut Butter	160	1 bar
Fiber One Oats and Chocolate	140	1 bar
Kellogg's Fiber Plus Antioxidants Dark Chocolate Almond	130	1 bar
Kellogg's Fiber Plus Antioxidants Chocolatey Peanut Butter	130	1 bar
Nature Valley Fruit & Nut Trail Mix Bar	140	1 bar
Nature Valley Oats 'n Dark Chocolate Crunchy Granola Bar	90	1 bar
Nature Valley Sweet & Salty Nut Almond Granola Bar	160	1 bar
Nature Valley Granola Nut Clusters Roasted Cashew	140	1 oz (about 7 clusters)

More *CarbLovers*-Approved Foods

The following foods are all rich in Resistant Starch or one of the other metabolism boosters recommended on *The CarbLovers Diet*.

RICH IN RESISTANT STARCH

Food	Calories	Serving Size
Aunt Millie's Healthy Goodness Fiber & Flavor Potato Bread	120	2 slices
Aunt Millie's Healthy Goodness Whole Grain White Bread	95	2 slices
Aunt Millie's Fiber for Life 12-Whole Grains Bread	110	1 slice
Aunt Millie's Healthy Goodness Light 5-Grain Bread	80	2 slices
Aunt Millie's Whole Grain Blueberry Muffins	170	1 muffin
Aunt Millie's Whole Grain Brownie Muffins	220	1 muffin
Aunt Millie's Whole Grain Chocolate Chip Muffins	190	1 muffin
Aunt Millie's Whole Grain Coffee Cake Muffins	190	1 muffin
Ener-G Foods Corn Loaf	40	1 slice
Ener-G Foods Seattle Brown Hamburger Buns & Hot Dog Buns	160	1 bun
Ener-G Foods Wylde Pretzels	130	40 pretzels
Ener-G Foods Brown Rice English Muffins (with Flax)	180	1 muffin
ExtendBar	150	1 bar
King Arthur Flour Hi-maize Natural Fiber (use in recipes)	15	1½ tbsp
King Arthur Flour Hi-maize High Fiber Flour (use in recipes)	90	¼ cup
Racconto Essentials Glycemic Health Whole Grain Pasta	170	2 oz
Wellness Bakeries Chocolate Bliss Cake Mix	178	$\frac{1}{12}$ of baked cake

RICH IN MONOUNSATURATED FATTY ACIDS (MUFAs)

Food	Calories	Serving Size
Olivio Premium Spread with Olive Oil	80	1 tbsp
Land O' Lakes Butter with Olive Oil	90	1 tbsp
Triscuit, Rosemary & Olive Oil Crackers	120	1 oz
Nature Valley Peanut Butter Granola Bars	190	2 bars
Hellmann's Mayonnaise with Olive Oil	50	1 tbsp
Kraft Mayo with Olive Oil	45	1 tbsp

RICH IN OMEGA-3s

Food	Calories	Serving Size
Nature's Path Flax Plus flakes cereal	110	¾ cup
Arnold Natural Flax & Fiber bread	100	1 slice
Eggland's Best Organic Eggs	70	1 large egg
Tropicana Healthy Heart Orange Juice with Omega-3	120	8 oz
Smart Balance Fat-Free Milk with Omega-3s and Vitamin E	120	1 cup
Quaker Fiber & Omega-3 Peanut Butter Chocolate Granola Bars	150	1 bar
Hodgson Mill Multi-grain Hot Cereal with Flaxseed and Soy	160	⅓ cup
Barilla Plus Pasta	210	2 oz
Ronzoni Healthy Harvest Pasta	180	2 oz
Mariani Enhanced Wellness Berry Thrive with Omega-3 Dried Fruit	140	¼ cup

RICH IN FIBER

Food	Calories	Serving Size
Kellogg's All-Bran Original Cereal	80	½ cup
Fiber One Original Cereal	60	½ cup
Kashi Good Friends Cereal	160	1 cup
Cascadian Farm Hearty Morning Fiber Cereal	200	¾ cup
Thomas' Hearty Grains Double Fiber, Honey Wheat English Muffins	120	1 muffin
Yoplait Fiber One Yogurt	50	1 (4 oz) container
Dannon Activia Fiber Yogurt	110	1 (4 oz) container
Kellogg's Fiber Plus Antioxidants Chocolate Chip Granola Bars	120	1 bar
Kellogg's Fiber Plus Antioxidants Dark Chocolate Almond Granola Bars	130	1 bar
Quaker Oatmeal-to-Go High Fiber Maple Brown Sugar	210	1 bar
Wheat Thins Fiber Selects	120	1 oz
Wasa Fiber Crispbread Crackers	30	1 slice
Ronzoni Smart Taste (3x the Fiber)	180	2 oz
Barilla Whole Grain Thin Spaghetti	200	2 oz
Mariani Enhanced Wellness Berry Defense Dried Fruit	130	¼ cup
Progresso High Fiber Minestrone Soup	110	1 cup
Arnold Natural Flax & Fiber Bread	100	1 slice

TOP RESISTANT STARCH FOODS

Food	Calories	Serving Size	Grams RS
Banana, green	105	1 medium (7–8")	12.5g
Banana, ripe	105	1 medium (7–8")	4.7g
Oatmeal, raw/cooked	153	½ cup	4.6g
Beans, white, cooked/canned	124	½ cup	3.8g
Lentils, cooked	115	½ cup	3.4g
Potatoes, cooked & cooled	118	1 potato; 2.5" diameter	3.2g
Plantain, cooked	89	½ cup, slices	2.7g
Beans, garbanzo, cooked/canned	143	½ cup	2.1g
Pasta, whole-wheat, cooked	174	1 cup	2.0g
Barley, pearled, cooked	97	½ cup	1.9g
Pasta, white, cooked & cooled	221	1 cup	1.9g
Beans, kidney, cooked/canned	112	½ cup	1.8g
Potatoes, boiled (skin & flesh)	118	1 potato	1.8g
Rice, brown, cooked	109	½ cup	1.7g
Beans, pinto, cooked/canned	122	½ cup	1.6g
Peas, vegetable/canned/frozen	62	½ cup	1.6g
Pasta, white, cooked	221	1 cup	1.5g
Beans, black, cooked/canned	114	½ cup	1.5g
Millet, cooked	104	½ cup	1.5g
Potatoes, baked (skin & flesh)	130	1 small	1.4g
Bread, pumpernickel	71	1 oz slice	1.3g
Corn polenta, cooked	113	½ cup	1.0g
Yam, cooked	79	½ cup cubes	1.0g
Potato chips	158	1 oz	1.0g
Cornflakes	100	1 cup	0.9g
Bread, rye (whole)	73	1 oz slice	0.9g
Puffed wheat	55	1¼ cup	0.9g
Crackers, rye crispbread	101	½ cup crushed	0.8g
Tortillas, corn	62	1 oz, 6" tortilla	0.8g
English muffin	134	1 whole muffin	0.7g
Bread, sourdough	82	1 oz slice "small"	0.6g
Crackers, rye crispbread	73	2 crispbreads	0.6g
Oatmeal, cooked	166	1 cup	0.5g
Bread, Italian	77	1 oz slice	0.3g
Bread, whole-grain	75	1 oz slice	0.3g
Corn chips	147	1 oz	0.2g
Crackers, crispbread (melba)	64	½ cup rounds	0.2g

TOP FIBER FOODS

The following foods are all naturally rich in fiber. Both the calorie and fiber amounts are given per 1-cup.

Food	Calories	Grams of Fiber
Artichokes	76	14g
Barley, pearled, cooked	193	6.0g
Beans, baked, canned	368	10g
Beans, black, cooked	228	15g
Beans, great northern, cooked	209	12g
Beans, kidney, cooked	225	11g
Beans, pinto, cooked	244	15g
Beans, navy, cooked	255	19g
Beans, white, cooked	299	13g
Buckwheat flour, whole-groat	402	12g
Bulgur, cooked	151	8g
Chickpeas (garbanzo beans), cooked	268	13g
Dates, chopped	415	12g
Lentils, cooked, boiled, without salt	230	16g
Lima beans, large, cooked	216	13 g
Oat bran, raw	231	15g
Peas, split, cooked	231	16g
Raspberries, frozen	64	11 g
Refried beans, canned, vegetarian	201	11 g
Soup, bean with ham, canned, chunky, ready-to-serve	231	11g
Wheat flour, whole-grain	407	15g

TOP MONOUNSATURATED FATTY ACIDS (MUFAS) FOODS

These foods are all naturally rich in MUFAs.

Food	Calories	Serving Size	MUFA
Avocados	322	1 avocado	20g
Macadamia nuts, dry roasted	203	1 oz (10–12 nuts)	16.8g
Semisweet chocolate chips	806	1 cup	16.7g
Hazelnuts or filberts	178	1 oz (21 nuts)	12.9g
Pecans	196	1 oz (20 halves)	11.6g
Pork, spareribs	337	3 oz	11.5g
Pork, ribs	314	3 oz	11.4g
Lamb, chops	305	3 oz	10.6g
Olive oil	119	1 tbsp	9.9g
Ricotta cheese	428	1 cup	8.9g
Canola oil	124	1 tbsp	8.9g
Almonds	163	1 oz (23 nuts)	8.8g
Salmon	335	½ fillet	8.2g
Cashews	163	1 oz	7.7g
Peanuts	166	1 oz (approx 28)	7.4g
Brazil nuts	186	1 oz (6–8 nuts)	7.0g
Pistachios	162	1 oz (49 nuts)	6.9g
Sunflower seed kernels	186	¼ cup	3.0g

TOP OMEGA-3 FOODS

These are the planet's richest foods in omega-3s, ranked from most to least.

Food	Calories	Serving Size	MUFA
Walnuts	185	1 oz	2.6g
Mackerel, canned, drained	177	4 oz	1.5g
Salmon	184	3 oz	1.2g
Tuna, canned	109	3 oz	0.7g
Fish, herring, Atlantic, kippered	62	1 oz	0.6g
Anchovies	60	1 oz	0.6g
Pollock	100	3 oz	0.5g
Flounder	99	3 oz	0.5g
Clams	126	3 oz	0.3g
Shrimp	84	3 oz	0.3g
Haddock	95	3 oz	0.2g
Catfish	89	3 oz	0.2g
Cod	89	3 oz	0.1g

Ask the carb pro

Frances Largeman-Roth, RD

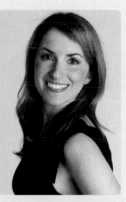

Q. Should I spread the word about carbs?

A. I like to think of carbs as my secret weapon. Wonder Woman's secret weapons are her indestructible bracelets and her lasso of truth. Mine is Resistant Starch. It can be your secret weapon, too! It's up to you whether you generously share it with friends or keep it to yourself. Either way, high-Resistant Starch carbs like bananas and oatmeal are your fabulous secret to fitting into that little black dress.

"I Lost Weight on *CarbLovers*"

BEFORE

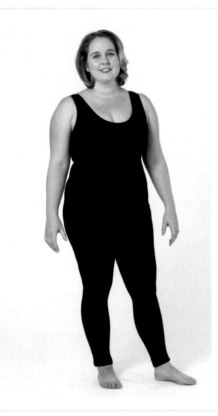

JENNIFER BERTSCH

Age: 38

Height: 5'5"

Weight before: 195

Weight after: 190

Pounds lost: 5

Biggest success moment: Losing 3 pounds in the first week, without feeling hungry.

Biggest challenge: Trying to convince my husband to eat the whole grains on *CarbLovers* was tricky!

Favorite recipe: Seared Chicken Breasts with French Potato Salad (page 185). It's ready in 35 minutes, and it is something my husband and I enjoy after work.

Even though I've always loved to cook—I trained as a pastry chef—my weight was under control until I moved from Montana to New York City. Working more than 40 hours a week made it harder to sneak in workouts, and the pounds quickly piled on. I have high blood pressure, and I knew, for my heart's sake, that I needed to clean up my diet. Of course, I wouldn't mind fitting in a size 10 again!

The emphasis on fresh food is what attracted me to *The CarbLovers Diet.* I knew I could stick to it because it focused on high-quality foods, like complex carbohydrates and fresh produce. It was also easy to adapt *CarbLovers* to my tastes. For example, I couldn't eat a whole banana in one sitting, so I began baking banana bread, using whole-wheat flour and natural sweeteners like honey. When we weren't in the mood for whole-grain products and fish, I swapped roasted, skinless chicken for shellfish, and snuck in sweet potatoes as a side dish.

Unlike other diets, I didn't feel like I was missing out on my favorite foods, and my energy levels were high enough to make me feel up for training for a 10K run. Though my weight loss has been slow and steady, I know that if I continue on *CarbLovers,* I'll be able to enjoy gourmet flavors while watching the pounds drop off.

Endnotes

CHAPTER 1

[1]Janine A. Higgins and others, "Resistant Starch Consumption Promotes Lipid Oxidation," *Nutrition & Metabolism,* 1, no. 8 (2004): 1-11.

[2]Janine A. Higgins, "Resistant Starch: Metabolic Effects and Potential Health Benefits," *Journal of AOAC International* 87, no. 3 (2004): 761-768.

[3]"Dietary Resistant Starch Increases Hypothalamic POMC Expression in Rats," *Obesity,* (Oct. 23, 2008): 1-9, doi:10.1038/oby.2008.483.

[4]Michael J. Keenan and others, "Effects of Resistant Starch, a Non-Digestible Fermentable Fiber, on Reducing Body Fat," *Obesity,* 14, no. 9 (2006): 1523-1534.

[5]Anwar T. Merchant and others, "Carbohydrate Intake and Overweight and Obesity among Healthy Adults," *Journal of the American Dietetic Association,* 109 (2009): 1165-1172.

[6]Mary M. Murphy, Judith Spungen Douglass, and Anne Birkett, "Resistant Starch Intakes in the United States," *Journal of the American Dietetic Association,* 108 (2008): 67-78.

CHAPTER 2

[1]Grant D. Brinkworth and others, "Long-Term Effects of a Very Low-Carbohydrate Diet and a Low-Fat Diet on Mood and Cognitive Function," *Archives of Internal Medicine,* 169, no. 20 (2009): 1873-1880.

[2]Jennifer S. Coelho, Janet Polivy, and C. Peter Herman, "Selective Carbohydrate or Protein Restriction: Effects on Subsequent Food Intake and Cravings," *Appetite,* 47 (2006): 352-360.

[3]Ilana Greenberg and others, "Adherence and Success in Long-Term Weight Loss Diets: The Dietary Intervention Randomized Controlled Trial," *Journal of the American College of Nutrition,* 28, no. 2 (2009): 159-169.

[4]William S. Yancy Jr. and others, "A Low-Carbohydrate, Ketogentic Diet versus a Low-Fat Diet to Treat Obesity and Hyperlipidemia," *Annals of Internal Medicine,* 140 (2004): 769-777.

[5]Jennifer S. Coelho, Janet Polivy, and C. Peter Herman, "Selective Carbohydrate or Protein Restriction: Effects on Subsequent Food Intake and Cravings," *Appetite,* 47 (2006): 352-360.

[6]Anwar T. Merchant and others, "Carbohydrate Intake and Overweight and Obesity among Healthy Adults," *Journal of the American Dietetic Association,* 109 (2009): 1165-1172.

[7]C. L. Bodinham, G. S. Frost, and M. D. Robertson, "The Acute Effects of Resistant Starch on Appetite and Satiety," *Proceedings of the Nutrition Society,* 67(May 2008): E157. Presented at the joint meeting of the Société Francaise de Nutrition and The Nutrition Society, 6-7 December 2007.

[8]Janine A. Higgins, "Resistant Starch: Metabolic Effects and Potential Health Benefits," *Journal of AOAC International* 87, no. 3 (2004): 761-768.

[9]Po-Wah So and others, "Impact of Resistant Starch on Body Fat Patterning and Central Appetite Regulation," *PLoS ONE,* 2, no. 12 (2007), http://www.plosone.org/article/info%3Adoi%2F10.1371%2Fjournal.pone.0001309.

[10]Po-Wah So and others, "Impact of Resistant Starch on Body Fat Patterning and Central Appetite Regulation," *PLoS ONE,* 2, no. 12 (2007), http://www.plosone.org/article/info%3Adoi%2F10.1371%2Fjournal.pone.0001309.

[11]Po-Wah So and others, "Impact of Resistant Starch on Body Fat Patterning and Central Appetite Regulation," *PLoS ONE,* 2, no. 12 (2007), http://www.plosone.org/article/info%3Adoi%2F10.1371%2Fjournal.pone.0001309.

[12]Janine A. Higgins and others, "Resistant Starch Consumption Promotes Lipid Oxidation," *Nutrition & Metabolism,* 1, no. 8 (2004): 1-11.

[13]Mary M. Murphy, Judith Spungen Douglass, and Anne Birkett, "Resistant Starch Intakes in the United States," *Journal of the American Dietetic Association,* 108 (2008): 67-78.

CHAPTER 3

[1]A. J. Hill and others, "Oral Administration of Proteinase Inhibitor II from Potatoes Reduces Energy Intake in Man," *Physiology and Behavior,* 48, no. 2 (1990): 241-6.

[2]L. A. Tucker and K. S. Thomas, "Increasing Total Fiber Intake Reduces Risk of Weight and Fat Gains in Women," *The Journal of Nutrition,* 139, no. 3 (2009): 576-581.

[3]Iris Shai and others, "Weight Loss with a Low-Carbohydrate, Mediterranean, or Low-Fat Diet," *The New England Journal of Medicine,* 259 (June 17, 2008): 229-241.

[4]Nicola M. McKeown and others, "Whole-Grain Intake and Cereal Fiber Are Associated with Lower Abdominal Adiposity in Older Adults," *The Journal of Nutrition*, 139, no. 10 (2009): 1950-1955.

[5]Morvarid Kabir and others, "Treatment for 2 mo with n-3 Polyunsaturated Fatty Acids Reduces Adiposity and Some Atherogenic Factors but Does Not Improve Insulin Sensitivity in Women with Type 2 Diabetes: A Randomized Controlled Study," *American Journal of Clinical Nutrition*, 86 (2007): 1670-1679.

[6]Lone G. Rasmussen and others, "Effect on 24-h Energy Expenditure of a Moderate-Fat Diet in Monounsaturated Fatty Acids Compared with That of a Low-Fat, Carbohydrate-Rich Diet: A 6 mo Controlled Dietary Intervention Trial," *American Journal of Clinical Nutrition*, 85, no. 4 (2007): 1014-1022.

[7]Juan A. Paniagua and others, "Monounsaturated Fat–Rich Diet Prevents Central Body Fat Distribution and Decreases Postprandial Adiponectin Expression Induced by a Carbohydrate-Rich Diet in Insulin-Resistant Subjects," *Diabetes Care*, 30, no. 7 (2007): 1717-1723.

[8]Carol S. Johnston, "Strategies for Healthy Weight Loss: From Vitamin C to the Glycemic Response," *Journal of the American College of Nutrition*, 24, no. 3 (2005): 158-165.

[9]Y. Wang and P. Jones, "Dietary Conjugated Linoleic Acid and Body Composition," *American Journal of Clinical Nutrition*, 79 (2004): 1153S-1158S.

[10]L. E. Norris and others, "Comparison of Dietary Conjugated Linoleic Acid with Safflower Oil on Body Composition in Obese Postmenopausal Women with Type 2 Diabetes Mellitus," *American Journal of Clinical Nutrition*, 90, no. 3 (2009): 468-476.

[11]R. N. Close and others, "Conjugated Linoleic Acid Supplementation Alters the 6-mo Change in Fat Oxidation During Sleep," *American Journal of Clinical Nutrition*, 86 (2007): 797-804.

[12]M. B. Zemel and others, "Dairy Augmentation of Total and Central Fat Loss in Obese Subjects," *International Journal of Obesity*, 29, vol. 4 (2005): 391-397.

CHAPTER 5

[1]L. E. Burke and others, "Using Instrumental Paper Diaries to Document Self-Monitoring Patterns in Weight Loss," *Contemporary Clinical Trials*, 29, no. 2 (2008): 182-193.

[2]L. E. Burke and others, "SMART Trial: A Randomized Controlled Clinical Trial of Self-Monitoring in Behavioral Weight Management-Design and Baseline Findings," *Contemporary Clinical Trials*, 30, no. 6 (2009): 540-551.

CHAPTER 7

[1]Yanni Papanikolaou and Victor L. Fulgoni, "Bean Consumption Is Associated with Greater Nutrient Intake, Reduced Systolic Blood Pressure, Lower Body Weight, and a Smaller Waist Circumference in Adults: Results from the National Health and Nutrition Examination Survey 1999-2002," *Journal of the American College of Nutrition*, 27, no. 5 (2008): 569-576.

[2]A. J. Hill and others, "Oral Administration of Proteinase Inhibitor II from Potatoes Reduces Energy Intake in Man," *Physiology and Behavior*, 48, no. 2 (1990):241-246.

[3]N. Schroeder and others, "Influence of Whole Grain Barley, Whole Grain Wheat, and Refined Rice-Based Foods on Short-Term Satiety and Energy Intake," *Appetite*, 53, no. 5 (2009): 363-369.

[4]Leonora N. Panlasigui and Lilian U. Thompson, "Blood Glucose Lowering Effects of Brown Rice in Normal and Diabetic Subjects," *International Journal of Food Science and Nutrition*, 57, no. 3-4 (2006): 151-158.

[5]Jung Yun Kim and others, "Meal Replacement with Mixed Rice Is More Effective than White Rice in Weight Control, While Improving Antioxidant Enzyme Activity in Obese Women," *Nutrition Research*, 28, no. 2 (2008): 66-71.

CHAPTER 8

[1]Barbara E. Kahn and Brian Wansink, "The Influence of Assortment Structure on Perceived Variety and Consumption Quantities," *Journal of Consumer Research*, 30, no. 4 (2004): 519.

[2]Mary M. Murphy, Judith Spungen Douglass, and Anne Birkett, "Resistant Starch Intakes in the United States," *Journal of the American Dietetic Association*, 108 (2008): 67-78.

[3]Snitker S, Fujishima Y, Shen H, Ott S, Pi-Sunyer X, Furuhata Y, Sato H, Takahashi M, "Effects of novel capsinoid treatment on fatness and energy metabolism in humans: possible pharmacogenetic implications," *American Journal of Clinical Nutrition* 2009 89 45-50.

[4]M. S. Westerterp-Plantenga, M. P. Lejeune, E. M. Kovacs, "Body Weight Loss and Weight Maintenance in Relations to Habitual Caffeine Intake and Green Tea Supplementation," *Obesity Research*, 13, no. 7 (2005): 1195-1204.

[5]Michelle C. Venables and others, "Green Tea Extract Ingestion, Fat Oxidation, and Glucose Tolerance in Healthy Humans," *American Journal of Clinical Nutrition*, 87, no. 3 (2008): 778-784.

[6]A. H. Eliasson and others, "Sleep Is a Critical Factor in the Maintenance of a Healthy Weight," Presented at the June 2009 SLEEP Conference.

[7]S. R. Patel and others, "Association Between Reduced Sleep and Weight Gain in Women," *American Journal of Epidemiology*, 164, no. 10 (2006): 947-954.

[8]J. E. Donnelly and others, "Appropriate Physical Activity Intervention Strategies for Weight Loss and Prevention of Weight Regain for Adults: American College of Sports Medicine Position Stand," *Medicine & Science in Sports & Exercise*, 41, no. 2 (2009): 459-471.

Recipe Index

Subject Index

Oxmoor House
VP, Publishing: Jim Childs
Editorial Director: Susan Payne Dobbs
Brand Manager: Fonda Hitchcock
Senior Editors: Heather Averett, Rebecca Brennan
Managing Editor: Laurie S. Herr

The CarbLovers Diet
Project Editor: Vanessa Lynn Rusch
Senior Designer: Emily Parrish
Director, Test Kitchens: Elizabeth Tyler Austin
Assistant Director, Test Kitchens: Julie Christopher
Test Kitchens Professionals: Allison E. Cox, Julie Gunter,
Kathleen Royal Phillips, Catherine Crowell Steele,
Ashley T. Strickland
Photography Director: Jim Bathie
Senior Photo Stylist: Kay E. Clarke
Associate Photo Stylist: Katherine Eckert Coyne
Production Manager: Theresa Beste-Farley

CONTRIBUTORS
Designer: Maxine Davidowitz
Compositor: Carol O. Loria
Photo Stylist: Mindy Shapiro
Copy Editor: Dolores Hydock
Fact Checkers: Jasmine Hodges, Carmine Loper
Proofreader: Norma Butterworth-McKittrick
Indexer: Nanette Cardon
Interns: Sarah M. Bélanger, Torie Cox,
Georgia Dodge, Perri Hubbard,
Allison Sperando

To order additional publications, call 1-800-765-6400.
For more books to enrich your life, visit **oxmoorhouse.com**